Acknowledgements:

Annette Snavely

Bing

Jacque and David

Nova

https://www.cakenknife.com/chipotle-chorizo-guacamole/

https://www.slurrp.com/recipes/banana-caramel-slice-1619713002

https://www.unconventionalbaker.com/raw-cherimoya-custard-fruit-sweetened-dairy-free/

https://www.foodfashionparty.com/2015/09/15/chocolate-coconut-ladoo/

https://sunkissedkitchen.com/dragon-fruit-smoothie/

https://www.bunsenburnerbakery.com/homemade-fig-bars/

https://mission-food.com/guava-bars/

https://www.recipestonourish.com/honeydew-melon-agua-fresca-with-lime/

https://www.food.com/recipe/kiwi-quick-bread-123565

https://www.bbcgoodfood.com/recipes/key-lime-pie-1

https://www.bbcgoodfood.com/recipes/refreshing-lychee-lime-sorbet

https://www.simplyrecipes.com/recipes/homemade_mango_chutney/

https://www.tasteofhome.com/recipes/orange-cheesecake-breakfast-rolls/

https://www.feastingathome.com/mexican-papaya-salad/

https://www.pinterest.es/pin/415949715559898347/ Little nectarine picnic cakes
https://en.petitchef.com/recipes/other/passionfruit-scones-fid-963388

https://www.tasteofhome.com/article/learning-how-to-make-meringue-we-reveal-our-secrets/

https://www.thespruceeats.com/baked-quince-recipe-2355425

https://suwanneerose.com/2016/12/star-fruit-chips/

https://cookpad.com/us/recipes/13601118-tamarind-baked-vegetables

https://www.bbcgoodfood.com/recipes/chilli-tangerine-braised-lentils

https://www.wellplated.com/watermelon-smoothie/

Tropical Superfruits of Mexico

Dedication to Christian Alejandro Haro Benavidez and the 50+ million visitors coming to Mexico this year.

Introduction:

If you are looking for a way to boost your health and vitality, you may want to explore the Tropical Superfruits of Mexico. These are fruits that have been used for centuries by the indigenous people of this diverse and colorful country, and that offer a range of benefits for your body and mind. Some other delectable, delicious items that originally grew in other tropical areas of the world have been imported and adopted into the culture, becoming additional providers of natural vitamins, nutrients, and antioxidants. The fertile soil of our Mexican land has aided in the production of all these fruits.

In this reference manual, you will discover twenty-four sensational superfruits that come from the tropical regions of Mexico: avocado, banana, cherimoya, coconut, dragon fruit, fig, guava, honeydew, jackfruit, kiwi, lime, lychee, mango, nectarine, oranges, papaya, passion fruit, pineapples, pomarosa, quince, starfruit, tamarind, tangerines, watermelon. You will learn about their description, their nutritional profiles, their health benefits, and how to use them in delicious recipes.

You will also find out how these superfruits can help you with various health issues, such as fatigue, inflammation, digestion, immunity, mood, skin, hair, and more. Whether you want to lose weight, gain energy, prevent disease, or simply enjoy a more balanced and vibrant lifestyle, this reference manual will show you how the tropical superfruits of Mexico can help you achieve your goals.

This reference manual is not only informative but also inspiring. It will take you on a journey through the rich history and culture of Mexico and show you how its people have harnessed the power of nature to nourish their bodies and souls. You will also get a glimpse of the beauty and diversity of Mexico's tropical landscapes, where these superfoods grow and thrive.

By reading this reference manual, you will gain a new appreciation for the tropical superfruits of Mexico, and how they can enhance your health and happiness. You will also discover a new way of eating that is delicious, satisfying, and good for you. So, get ready to explore the tropical superfruits of Mexico, and enjoy the journey!

Index:

- Avocado
- Banana
- Cherimoya
- Coconut
- Dragon fruit
- Fig
- Guava
- Honeydew
- Jackfruit
- Kiwi
- Lime
- Lychee
- Mango
- Nectarine
- Oranges
- Papaya
- Passion fruit
- Pineapples
- Pomarosa
- Quince
- Star fruit
- Tamarind
- Tangerines
- Watermelon

For good reason, tropical fruits have been treasured for ages. They are a well-liked addition to many cuisines all over the world because of their amazing flavors and health advantages. We hope that after reading this guide you will have a renewed respect for the wide variety of tropical fruits.

So why not experiment and do something different, like incorporating a tropical fruit into your regular smoothie or using it to make a delicious dessert? There is no excuse not to enjoy these delectable and healthy fruits given the limitless possibilities.

FRUIT FAST

You may think that eating fruit simply means buying fruit, chopping it up and putting it in your mouth.

It's not as easy as that. It's important to know how and *when* to eat fruit.

What is the right way to eat fruit?

IT IS NOT EATING FRUIT AFTER YOUR MEAL

WE SHOULD EAT FRUIT DURING A FAST

Eating fruit while fasting will play a major role in detoxifying your system while giving you a lot of energy in your weight loss efforts as well as in other life activities.

FRUIT IS THE CRITICAL COMPONENT!

Let's say you eat two slices of bread and then one slice of fruit.

While the slice of fruit is ready to go directly into the intestines through the stomach, it is prevented because of the bread you ate before the fruit!

Meanwhile, the whole meal consisting of bread and fruit decomposes, ferments, and becomes acidic. As soon as fruit encounters food and digestive secretions in the stomach, all the food mass (everything) begins to decompose.

Here is why acidic conditions can be bad.

Bloating: One common reaction to fermented foods is a temporary increase in gas and bloating. This occurs because probiotics, the beneficial microorganisms found in fermented foods, kill harmful gut bacteria and fungi. As a result, excess gas is produced during this process. While some bloating is a sign that harmful bacteria are being removed from the gut, severe bloating can be uncomfortable and painful.

Headaches and Migraines: Fermented foods naturally contain biogenic amines, which are produced during the fermentation process. These amines are created by certain bacteria as they break down amino acids in the food. Unfortunately, for some individuals, these biogenic amines can trigger headaches and migraines.

Acidic Environment: When fermented foods are present in the stomach, they introduce additional acids. While some acids are beneficial (such as those produced by probiotics), an excessively acidic environment can potentially irritate the stomach lining. This irritation may lead to symptoms like heartburn or discomfort.

Therefore, please eat your fruit while fasting or before your meals!

You have probably heard people complain:

"Every time I eat watermelon, I burp; if I eat a banana, I feel like going to the bathroom, etc...", etc.... ".

This won't happen if you eat fruit while fasting!

Fruit mixes with the decomposition of other foods, and gases, hence the belly bloating!

Graying hair, baldness, nervous breakdowns, under-eye circles: all these things have less chance or happening if you fruit fast.

There is no fruit as sour as orange and lemon, and all fruits become alkaline in our bodies, according to Dr. Herbert Shelton, an American naturopath, alternative medicine advocate, author, pacifist, vegan, and a supporter of rawist and fasting.

If you've mastered the right way to eat fruits, you already have the SECRET of beauty, longevity, health, energy, happiness, and normal weight.

If you need to drink juice, drink fresh juice, and NOT juice from cans, packets, or bottles!

Especially don't drink warm juice.

Don't eat prepared fruits (cooked, boiled) because you won't have all the nutrients. You will only get a taste of it. Cooking destroys all vitamins! Eating the whole fruit is better than drinking the juice.

If you wish to drink fresh fruit juice, drink it slowly, sip by sip so it can mix with your saliva before swallowing it.

You can do a 3-day fruit fast to cleanse or detoxify your body.

Eat nothing but fruit and drink nothing but fruit juice for 3 days. You'll be surprised when your friends tell you how better you look!

KIWI FRUIT: Very small but mighty.

It's a good source of potassium, magnesium, vitamin E, and fiber. It has twice as much vitamin C as an orange.

ORANGE: the most delicious medicine.

Eating 2-4 oranges a day will help keep colds away, lower cholesterol, and dissolve kidney stones. It will also help reduce the risk of colon cancer.

One of the tastiest, refreshing fruits is Watermelon. Consisting of 92% water, watermelon is also loaded with a high dose of glutathione, which helps us boost our immune system. Watermelon is a good source of lycopene, an oxidant to fight cancer. Vitamin C and potassium are other nutrients found in watermelon.

GUAVA AND PAPAYA:

These fruits are loaded with vitamin C. They deserve special recognition.

Guava is also rich in fiber, which helps prevent constipation.

Papaya is rich in carotene, which is good for your eyes.

DRINKING WATER

You may like to drink cold water or cold drinks.

However, cold water or cold drink will solidify the oily or fatty matter that you just ate.

This will slow down digestion.

Once this mixture reacts on contact with stomach acid, it will decompose and be absorbed by the intestines faster than solid meals.

This will carpet (solidify) the inside of the intestines.

Very soon it will turn into fat!

It's much better to have hot soup or drink hot water after eating.

Let's be careful and stay aware. The more we know, the better our chance of survival.

CONSUMING THE FRUITS WHILE FASTING

This message may open your eyes!

Dr. Stephen Mack of Baylor College of Medicine treats end-stage cancer patients in an "unorthodox" manner, and many patients have recovered their health.

Previously, he used solar energy to treat illness of his patients; he believes in the process of natural healing of diseases affecting the human body.

It's one of the strategies to cure cancer.

Cancer patients need not die. Indeed, we've already found the way to cure cancer: it's the way we eat fruit.

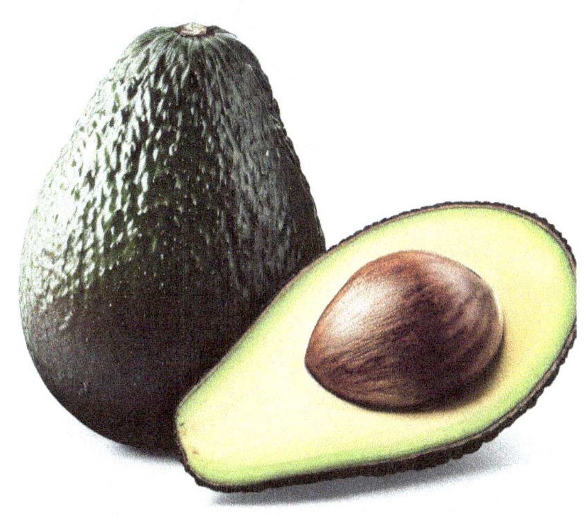

Avocado: a fruit that is quite popular because of its tasty texture and rich taste. This native is a common ingredient in guacamole, smoothies, and salads, among other dishes.

Avocados are not only tasty but also loaded with monounsaturated fats, fiber, and a variety of vitamins and minerals. Additionally, these luscious fruits include phytochemicals with anti-inflammatory and antioxidant properties.

The avocado is a medium-sized, evergreen tree in the laurel family. It is native to the Americas and was first domesticated by Mesoamerican tribes more than 5,000 years ago. Then, as now, it was prized for its large and unusually oily fruit. The fruit of domestic varieties have smooth, buttery, golden-green flesh when ripe. Depending on the cultivar, avocados have green, brown, purplish, or black skin, and may be pear-shaped, egg-shaped, or spherical.

For commercial purposes the fruits are picked while unripe and ripened after harvesting. The nutrient density and extremely high fat content of avocado flesh are useful to a variety of cuisines and are often eaten to enrich vegetarian diets.

Mexico's national fruit is avocado. Avocados first appeared in Mexico and Central America. When eating at a Mexican restaurant it is often enjoyed with mariachi bands and a waiter making guacamole at your table. It is an event that makes for a wonderful vacation memory.

Avocados are believed to have originated around 10,000 years ago in the tropical climates of Mexico, Guatemala, and the West Indies.

Peak avocado season is late winter and early spring.

The most readily available variety of avocado is Hass, also called avocado pear or alligator pear.

Avocado is actually a fruit, not a vegetable.

Avocados contain more fat than any other fruit or vegetable. Also, the trees contain enzymes that prevent the fruit from ever ripening on the tree, allowing farmers to use the trees as storage devices for up to 7 months after they reach full maturity, allowing avocados to always be in season.

Avocado extract may help relieve arthritic pain.

Avocado oil may accelerate wound healing.

Legend has it that a Japanese chef working in California in the 1960s once resorted to using avocado when he couldn't source tuna. The now extremely popular California Roll was born.

Avocado Recipe:

Chorizo & Creamy Guacamole

Ingredients:

2 x 200g bags salted tortilla chips

180g bag grated Monterey Jack cheese

1-2 jalapeño chiles, thinly sliced (deseeded if you don't like it too hot)

For the pickled onion salsa:

2 tbsp white wine vinegar or cider vinegar

1 tbsp sugar

1 red onion halved and finely sliced

2 tomatoes, seeds removed, cut into small pieces

3 radishes thinly sliced

For the chorizo beans:

1 tbsp olive oil

1 red onion finely chopped

2 x 60g packs cubed chorizo

400g can black beans, drained

2 tsp smoked paprika

2 tsp clear honey or agave syrup

For the creamy guacamole:

3 ripe avocados

zest and juice 1 large lime

handful cilantro, chopped, plus a few leaves to garnish

150g crema

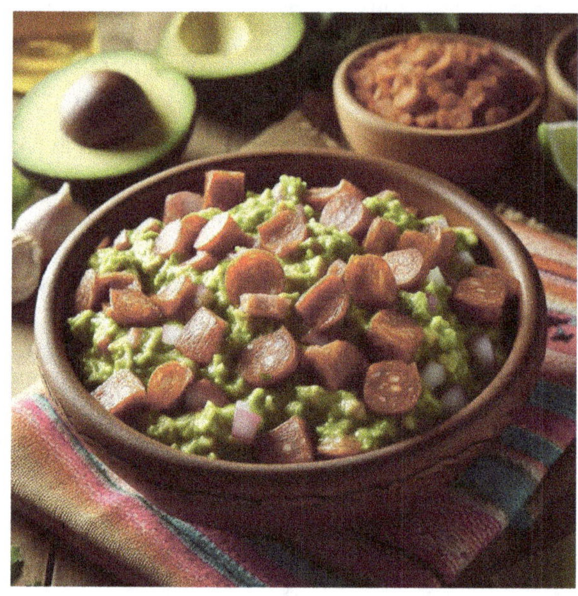

Method:

STEP 1

First, make the pickled onions for the salsa. Mix the vinegar, sugar, and 1 /2 tsp flaky sea salt in a bowl, whisking until the sugar and salt have dissolved. Add the onion, mix well, and set aside for 20 minutes, tossing around in the vinegar every few minutes.

STEP 2

Next, make the beans. Heat the oil in a frying pan, add the onion and cook gently for a few minutes until softened. Add the chorizo and cook for 2-3 minutes more, stirring until the oils have released into the pan. Add the beans and sizzle for a couple of minutes until softened a little. Sprinkle in the paprika, drizzle in the honey, cook for a few more minutes, then set aside.

STEP 3

To make the guacamole, halve two of the avocados and remove the stones. Slide a dessert spoon between the skin and the flesh of each avocado half and scoop the flesh into a bowl. Add the lime zest and half the juice, the cilantro, half the crema and a pinch of salt. Mash well until you have smooth guacamole, then cover and chill until ready to serve. Halve the remaining avocado and remove the stone. Cut the flesh in a crisscross pattern, then scoop out the chunks with a spoon and toss through the remaining lime juice.

STEP 4

Heat oven to 200c/395f. In your largest roasting tin or a large ovenproof dish, layer the tortilla chips, chorizo beans, cheese, and most of the chile slices. Bake for 10-15 minutes until the cheese has melted and the tortilla chips are toasted at the edges.

STEP 5

While the nachos are cooking, finish the salsa. Drain most of the pickling liquid from the onions and add the tomatoes, and radishes and toss together. Remove the nachos from the oven and scatter the salsa over them. Spoon on the guacamole, then scatter over the chunks of avocado. Mix the remaining crema with 2-3 tsp water until it's runny enough to drizzle over the nachos, and finish with extra chile if you like it hot. Finally, scatter with the remaining cilantro. Serve as soon as possible, with plenty of napkins!

Chorizo & Creamy Guacamole

Nutrition Facts

Servings: 12

Amount per serving

Calories	**318**

	% Daily Value*
Total Fat 23.3g	**30%**
Saturated Fat 8.6g	**43%**
Cholesterol 36mg	**12%**
Sodium 432mg	**19%**
Total Carbohydrate 18.5g	**7%**
Dietary Fiber 6.1g	**22%**
Total Sugars 5.1g	
Protein 11.4g	
Vitamin D 0mcg	0%
Calcium 159mg	12%
Iron 2mg	9%
Potassium 534mg	11%

*The % Daily Value (DV) tells you how much a nutrient in a food serving contributes to a daily diet. 2,000 calorie a day is used for general nutrition advice.

Recipe analyzed

by **very**well

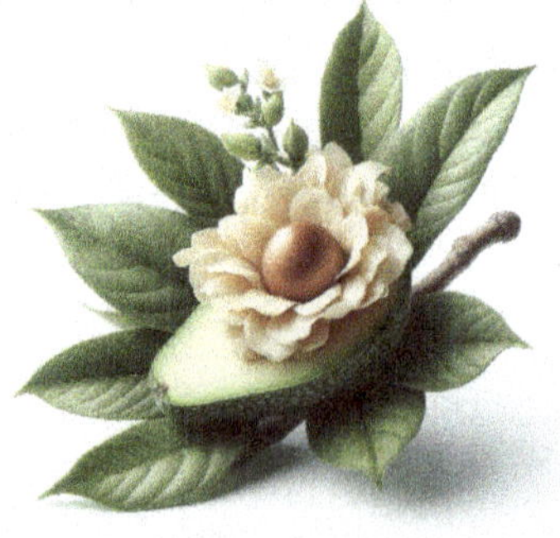

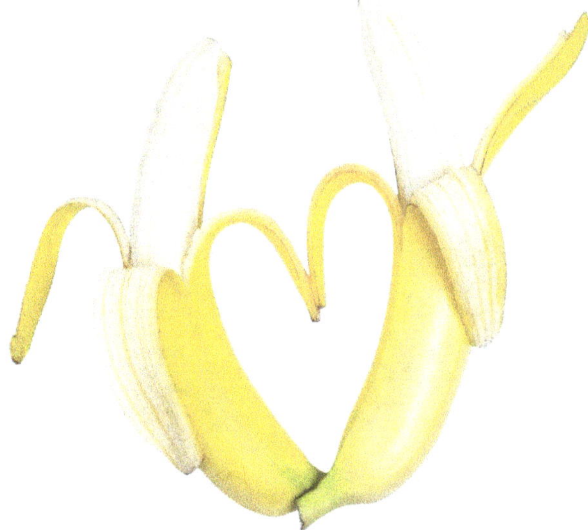

 a popular fruit consumed all over the world, loved for their high potassium, dietary fiber, and vitamin C content. Because of their inherent sweetness, they work great when sliced and added to cereal or yogurt for a quick and wholesome snack.

Bananas also perform well as a natural sweetener in baked goods and smoothies. They are a good substitute for eggs.

Bananas have great versatility and a complimentary flavor used in many different cuisines and dishes, from curry to ice cream. Here are some interesting facts about bananas that you may not have known:

The banana fruit got its name after being sold wrapped in aluminum foil for 10 cents at the 1876 Philadelphia World Fair.

In the past the classic banana species we consumed was called Gros Michel. It was a sweeter and creamier alternative to the modern banana. Due to a sweeping and catastrophic disease in 1965 across Central and Southern America, the farmers swapped to the modern variety.

There are over 1000 different varieties of bananas growing around the world, subdivided into 50 groups. Some are sweet, like the Cavendish bananas, which are the most common and most widely exported.

The banana is scientifically a berry, whereas the strawberry is not. This comes down to the classification of a berry. A berry must contain seeds inside the flesh, not outside.

If a person is allergic to bananas, or even avocados and chestnuts, they have an increased risk of being allergic to latex. Some say half of those allergic to latex are often allergic to bananas. This is due to the proteins within the banana.

A U.S. study found that bananas can help lower your risk of stroke and heart attack due to the level of potassium they contain. They do this by lowering the risk of stiffness in the aorta and hardening in the arteries.

Bananas Recipe:

Banana Caramel Slice

Ingredients:

2 (500g each) pkt banana & walnut bread slices

1/4 cup brown sugar, firmly packed

1/2 cup honey

395g can condensed milk

1 tsp vanilla extract

180g butter

100g dark chocolate, chopped

STEP 1

Grease a 20 x 30cm slice pan and line the base and sides with parchment paper. Trim the banana and walnut bread slices and place in the base of the pan to fit snugly.

STEP 2

Combine the sugar, honey, condensed milk, vanilla and 150g of the butter in a heavy-based saucepan over low heat. Cook, stirring, for 3-4 minutes or until sugar dissolves. Increase heat to medium-low. Cook, stirring, for 15-20 minutes or until mixture thickens and turns golden caramel.

STEP 3

Remove the caramel from the heat. Set aside to cool, stirring often, for 3-4 minutes. Pour the caramel over the banana bread and use a spatula to spread evenly. Set aside to cool completely.

STEP 4

Place the chocolate and remaining butter in a heatproof bowl. Microwave on High for 45 seconds to 1 minute or until melted and smooth. Spread evenly over the caramel. Garnish the top with banana half slices and chocolate bits. Place in the fridge for 15-20 minutes to set. Remove from the pan and cut into pieces.

Banana Nutritional Facts:

Banana Caramel Slice

Nutrition Facts

Servings: 6

Amount per serving

Calories	**1198**

	% Daily Value*
Total Fat 84.5g	**108%**
Saturated Fat 25.4g	**127%**
Cholesterol 91mg	**30%**
Sodium 276mg	**12%**
Total Carbohydrate 96.6g	**35%**
Dietary Fiber 8.4g	**30%**
Total Sugars 77.1g	
Protein 27.7g	
Vitamin D 17mcg	84%
Calcium 303mg	23%
Iron 4mg	21%
Potassium 1110mg	24%

The % Daily Value (DV) tells you how much a nutrient in a food serving contributes to a daily diet. 2,000 calorie a day is used for general nutrition advice.

Recipe analyzed

by **verywell**

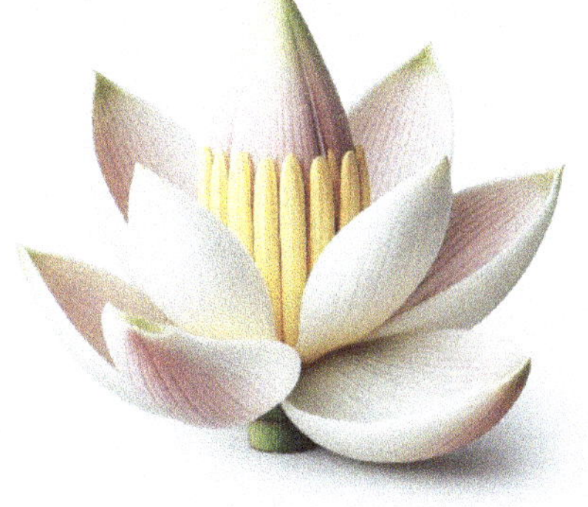

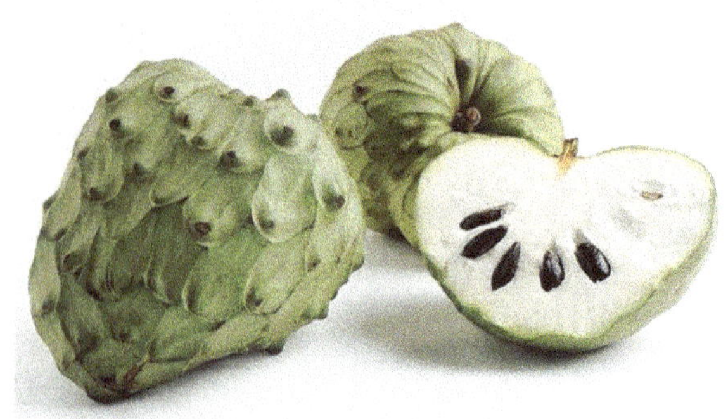

Cherimoya: tropical fruit cherimoya, which is also known as the "custard apple," is from South America and Mexico. This fruit is a treat to the taste buds thanks to its creamy texture and distinct flavor, which some people have compared to a combination of pineapple and banana.

Cherimoya is a member of the Annonacin family. Here are some interesting facts about cherimoya:

Mark Twain called the cherimoya, "the most delicious fruit known to men".

Cherimoya is a low-fat fruit that provides fiber and numerous micronutrients. The fruit is an excellent source of vitamin C and vitamin B6. It is also a good source of iron, riboflavin, and thiamin.

A single one-cup serving of cherimoya fruit (160 grams) provides about 120 calories, 1.1g of fat, 28.3g of carbohydrate, and 2.5g of protein.

Cherimoya is generally thought to be native to Colombia, Ecuador, Peru, and Bolivia, although it's spreading through cultivation to the Andes and Central America.

Cherimoya trees can grow up to 35 feet tall and produce fruit for up to 20 years.

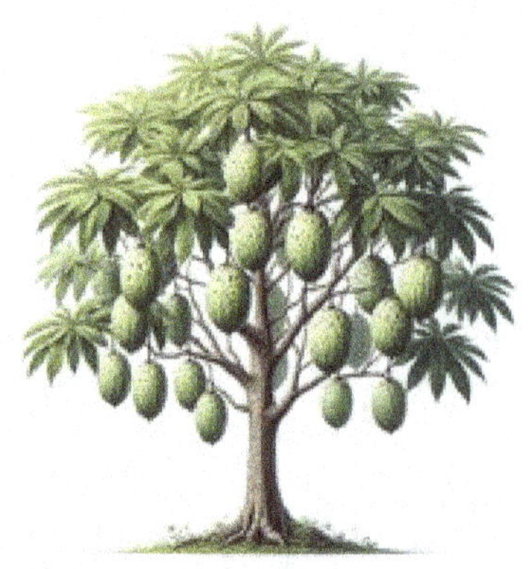

Cherimoya Recipe:

Raw Cherimoya Custard Pudding

Ingredients:

flesh of 1 ripe cherimoya (discard skin and seeds)

⅓ cup unsweetened vanilla almond milk

dash of salt

2 tbsp chopped pistachios

Instructions:

Blend all ingredients, except pistachios, into a smooth texture.

Transfer into a glass jar, and cover.

Chill in the freezer for about an hour, stir in pistachios, and enjoy!

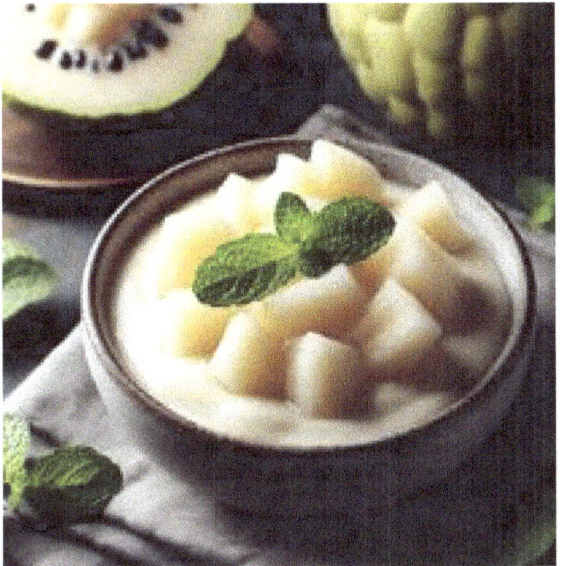

Raw Cherimoya Custard Pudding

Nutrition Facts	
Servings: 6	
Amount per serving	
Calories	**47**
	% Daily Value*
Total Fat 1.1g	**1%**
Saturated Fat 0.1g	**0%**
Cholesterol 0mg	**0%**
Sodium 46mg	**2%**
Total Carbohydrate 9.6g	**4%**
Dietary Fiber 1.4g	**5%**
Total Sugars 7.1g	
Protein 1.2g	
Vitamin D 0mcg	0%
Calcium 31mg	2%
Iron 0mg	1%
Potassium 163mg	3%

*The % Daily Value (DV) tells you how much a nutrient in a food serving contributes to a daily diet. 2,000 calorie a day is used for general nutrition advice.

Recipe analyzed

verywell

by

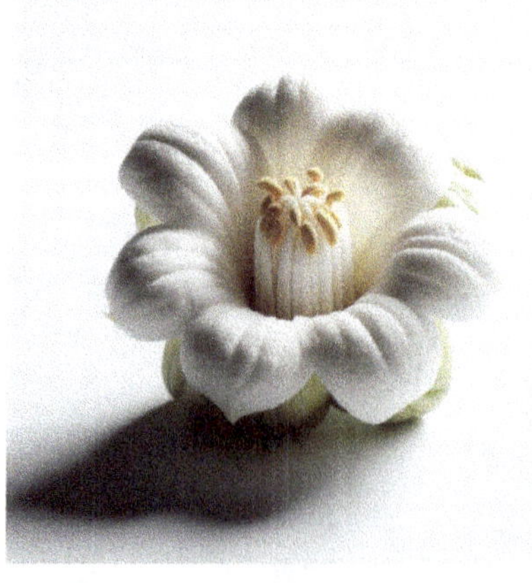

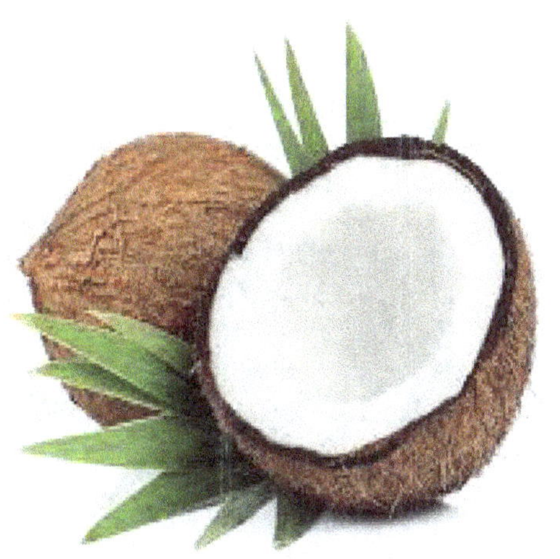

Coconut: a fruit that can be used in many ways in tropical cuisine. Its milk and oil are frequently used as the base for stews and sauces, while the flesh can be shredded and utilized in baking and cooking.

Young coconut water is a favorite beverage because it contains electrolytes and vitamins. Coconut oil is utilized for more than just cooking; it also helps to maintain healthy skin and hair.

Coconuts are a fascinating fruit that have been used for centuries in many different cultures. Here are some interesting facts about coconuts:

The name coconut is a combination of nut, and the Portuguese word coco, after the face-like image the shell has with the 3 holes.

Coconuts are not nuts but are classified as drupes. A drupe is a fruit that has a fleshy outer layer surrounding a hard pit or shell containing the seed.

Coconuts are an excellent source of fiber, potassium, manganese, and selenium.

Coconut water is a natural electrolyte and is rich in potassium, magnesium, and calcium. It is also low in calories and fat-free.

The coconut palm tree can grow up to 82 feet (25 meters) high and can produce up to 180 coconuts during a single harvest.

Coconuts have been used for many different purposes throughout history. For example, people have used coconut fibers to construct robust armor, and the husk of a coconut can be burnt to act as a natural mosquito repellent.

In 2022, there were over 62 million tons of coconuts produced worldwide.

An urban legend says that falling coconuts cause death. You can jump away from a snake, and you can step on a spider, but... you do not see or hear a coconut falling from a tree. Jeje!

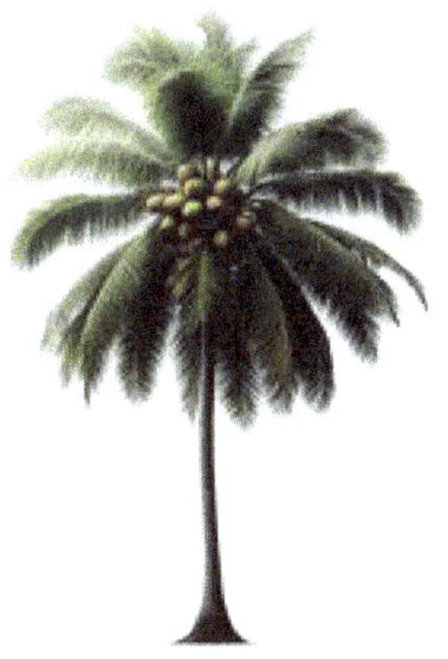

Coconut Recipe:

COCONUT-CASHEW-CHOCOLATE FUDGE/LADOO

Ingredients:

1 tbsp butter

2 cups cashew powder (not too fine, keep it coarse)

2 cups desiccated dry unsweetened coconut powder

⅓ cup condensed milk

⅓ tsp cardamom powder

a pinch of saffron strands

2 tsp raw cocoa powder

2 tsp melted milk chocolate

Some desiccated coconut to sprinkle on the fudge

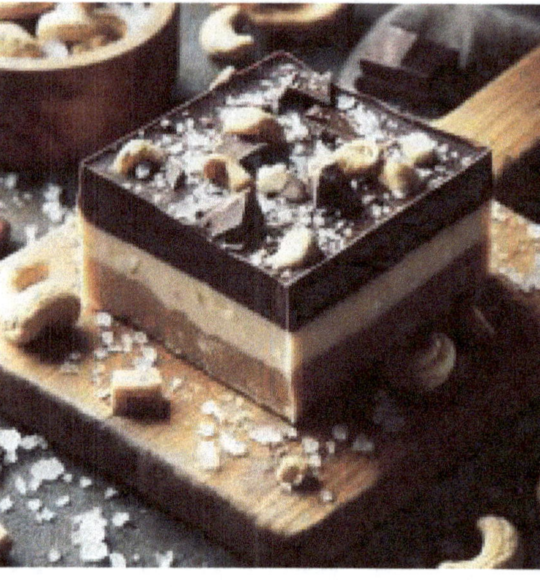

Instructions:

Heat a nonstick pan. Add the butter and let it melt on low to medium heat. Add the powdered cashews and keep stirring to toast everything. Do not brown it. Toast for 3-4 minutes.

Add the coconut powder, condensed milk and stir well to incorporate and cook for another 3-4 minutes on low heat.

Take the pan off the heat and add the cardamom, saffron strands and mix well.

Add the cocoa powder and milk chocolate and mix very well.

Spread in a baking pan and sprinkle with some desiccated coconut.

Stays good for 10 days in an airtight container, you could refrigerate it too. Just bring it to room temperature before serving.

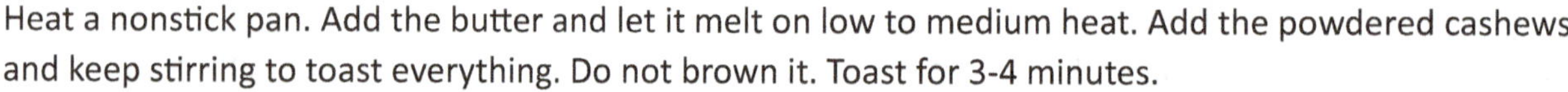

Coconut Nutritional Facts:

COCONUT-CASHEW-CHOCOLATE FUDGE/LADOO

Nutrition Facts

Servings: 6

Amount per serving

Calories	**437**

	% Daily Value*
Total Fat 34g	**44%**
Saturated Fat 14.5g	**73%**
Cholesterol 11mg	**4%**
Sodium 334mg	**15%**
Total Carbohydrate 29.6g	**11%**
Dietary Fiber 4.2g	**15%**
Total Sugars 13.8g	
Protein 9.5g	
Vitamin D 1mcg	7%
Calcium 75mg	6%
Iron 7mg	37%
Potassium 442mg	9%

*The % Daily Value (DV) tells you how much a nutrient in a food serving contributes to a daily diet. 2,000 calorie a day is used for general nutrition advice.

Recipe analyzed

by **very**well

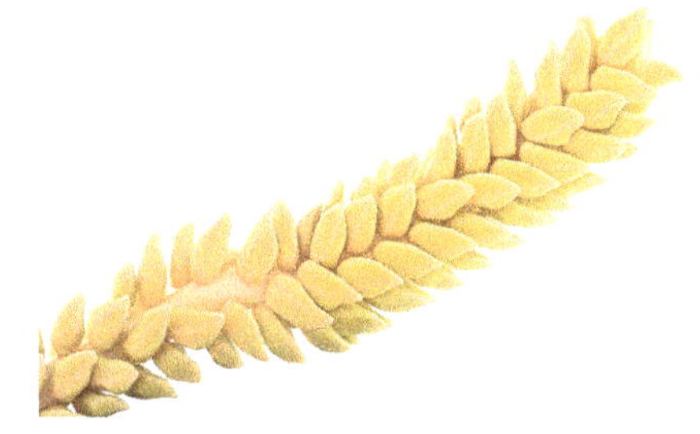

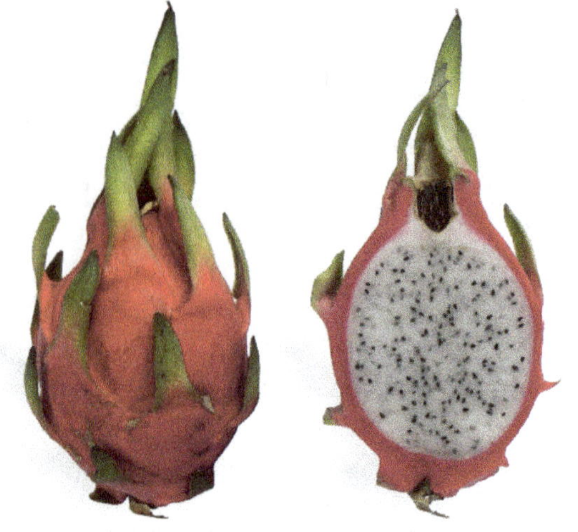

interesting facts about dragon fruit:

Dragon fruit grows on the Hylocereus cactus, also known as the Honolulu queen, whose flowers only open at night. The plant is native to southern Mexico and Central America. Today, it is grown all over the world.

The two most common types of dragon fruit have bright red skin with green scales that resemble a dragon — hence the name. The most widely available variety has white pulp with black seeds, though a less common type with red pulp and black seeds exists as well. Another variety — referred to as yellow dragon fruit — has yellow skin and white pulp with black seeds.

Dragon fruit is a low-calorie fruit that is high in fiber and provides a good number of vitamins and minerals. A single one-cup serving of dragon fruit (160 grams) provides about 60 calories, 1.2g of protein, 13 grams of carbohydrates, and 3 grams of fiber.

Dragon fruit is also a decent source of iron and magnesium. Given the high amount of fiber and magnesium, as well as the extremely low-calorie content, dragon fruit can be considered a highly nutrient-dense fruit.

Dragon fruit contains several types of antioxidants. These are compounds that protect your cells from unstable molecules called free radicals, which are linked to chronic diseases and aging. These are some of the main antioxidants contained in dragon fruit pulp:

Betalains: Found in the pulp of red dragon fruit, these deep red pigments have been shown to protect "bad" LDL cholesterol from becoming oxidized or damaged.

Hydroxycinnamates: This group of compounds has demonstrated anticancer activity in test-tube and animal studies.

Flavonoids: This large, diverse group of antioxidants is linked to better brain health and a reduced risk of heart disease.

Dragon Fruit Recipe:

Dragon Fruit Smoothie

Ingredients:

¾ cup mango chunks fresh or frozen

¾ cup dragon fruit

1 banana fresh or frozen - you can slice up a banana and freeze the slices on a tray then put in freezer bag until needed

¼ cup blueberries fresh or frozen

½ tbsp lime juice

¼ cup milk, almond or as you prefer

½ tbsp chia seeds plus another 1 tsp for garnish

Instructions:

Place all ingredients in a blender and blend until smooth.

Pour into a glass and top with some additional chia seeds, blueberries, or a few small chunks or slices of dragon fruit and mango.

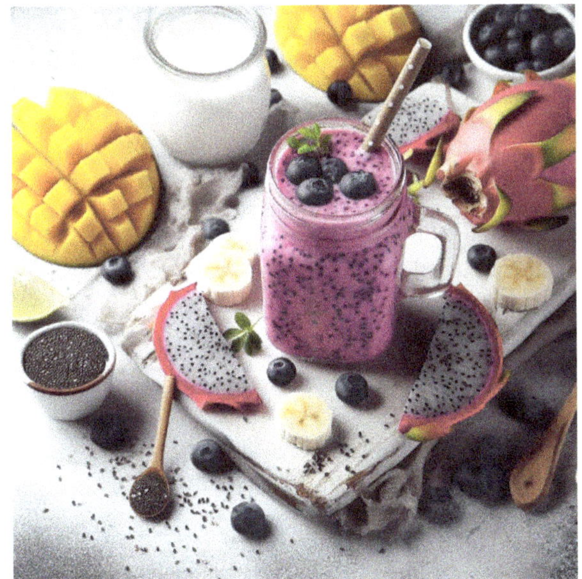

Dragon Fruit Nutritional Facts:

Dragon Fruit Smoothie

Nutrition Facts

Servings: 1

Amount per serving

Calories	**284**

	% Daily Value*
Total Fat 3.5g	**4%**
Saturated Fat 1.1g	**5%**
Cholesterol 5mg	**2%**
Sodium 39mg	**2%**
Total Carbohydrate 66.1g	**24%**
Dietary Fiber 7.3g	**26%**
Total Sugars 47.1g	
Protein 5.4g	
Vitamin D 0mcg	2%
Calcium 125mg	10%
Iron 1mg	7%
Potassium 744mg	16%

*The % Daily Value (DV) tells you how much a nutrient in a food serving contributes to a daily diet. 2,000 calorie a day is used for general nutrition advice.

Recipe analyzed by **verywell**

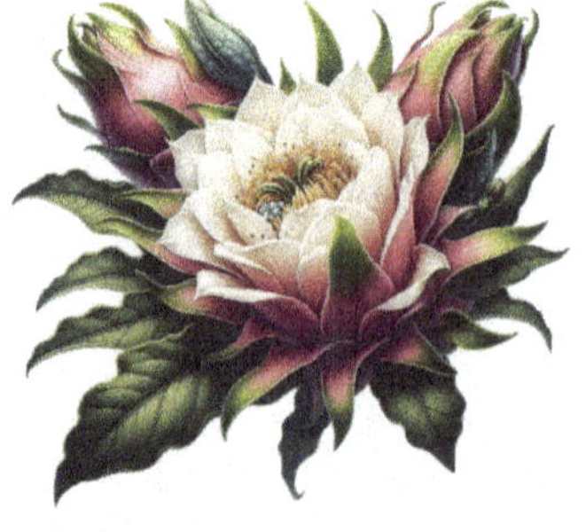

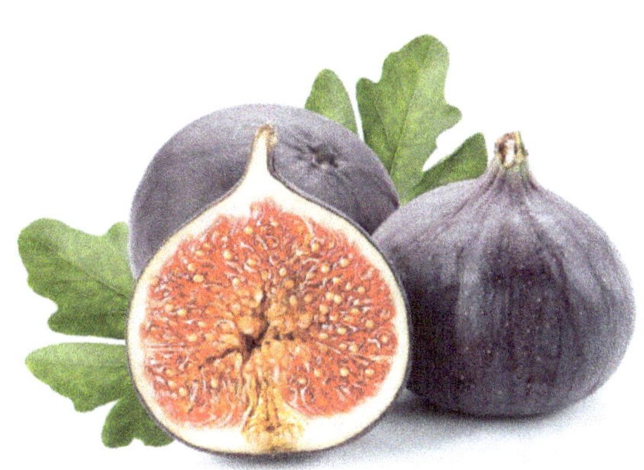

Fig: a fruit that comes from a tree that was one of the first to be cultivated in history. It is harvested from July through September. The black fig was originally brought from Spain and quickly found its home in the tropics.

Figs are a sweet fruit that is enjoyed by many people around the world. Here are some interesting facts about figs:

Figs are one of the oldest fruits in the world, with evidence of their cultivation dating back to 5,000 BC.

Figs are a good source of fiber and are rich in vitamins and minerals, including potassium, calcium, magnesium, iron, and copper. Figs also contain small amounts of a wide variety of nutrients, but they're particularly rich in copper and vitamin B6. Copper is a vital mineral that's involved in several bodily processes, including metabolism and energy production, as well as the formation of blood cells, connective tissues, and neurotransmitters. Vitamin B6 is a key vitamin necessary to help your body break down dietary protein and create new proteins. It also plays an important role in brain health. Figs have been used for centuries for their medicinal properties. They have been used to treat a variety of ailments, including constipation, bronchitis, and diabetes.

Figs are a popular ingredient in many different cuisines around the world. They can be eaten fresh or dried and are often used in desserts, jams, and chutneys.

Note: dried figs are high in sugar and rich in calories, as the sugar becomes concentrated when the fruits are dried.

The fig tree is a symbol of abundance, fertility, and sweetness.

There are over 750 known species of figs in the world, native across the globe. Nearly every species of fig tree is pollinated by its own distinct species of fig wasp. Although the average female fig wasp is only about 1.5 millimeters long, it plays a crucial role in the life cycle of the fig tree. Without the fig wasp, the fig tree would not be able to reproduce.

Another fig comes from the Higuera tree. It is plucked from the branches by birds and taken to their nests in nearby palm trees. The seeds are so small that they are not digested and are defecated as natural compost. The seeds sprout into vines that grow down from the top of the palm. Part way down the vines branch off and sprout leaves to aid in capturing sunlight to further its growth as it reaches for the soil. The tree leaves do not obscure the sunlight from the palm frowns. Once the vines absorb nutrients from the soil, the vines expand and become a tree encircling the palm. The Higuera takes some nutrients from the palm, but unlike its name "strangling fig", the Higuera coexists with the palm for hundreds of years. The older palm dies of old age and the Higuera continues as a majestic tree in the jungle.

Fig Recipe:

Fig Bars

Ingredients:

<u>For the crust</u>:

½ cup butter, softened

¼ cup sugar

½ teaspoon vanilla

1 cup all-purpose flour

<u>For the filling</u>:

¼ cup sugar

1 cup boiling water

1 cup dried figs chopped

<u>For the topping</u>:

¼ cup all-purpose flour

¼ cup packed brown sugar

3 tbsp cold butter

¼ cup quick-cooking oats

¼ cup chopped walnuts

Instructions:

Preheat oven to 175c/350f.

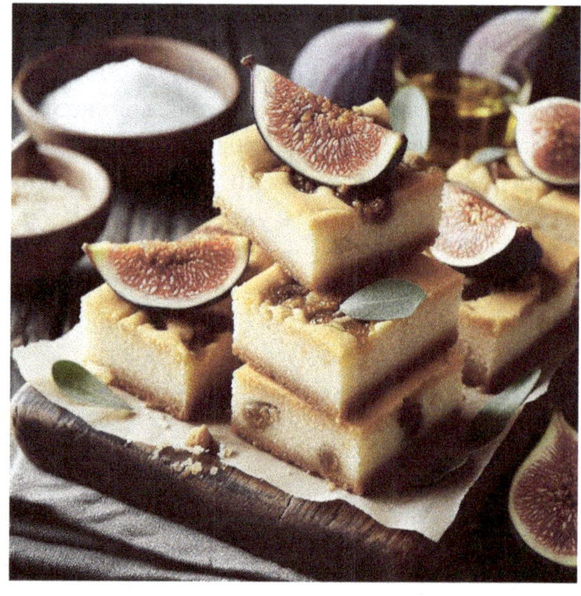

Spray a 9-inch square pan with cooking spray.

In small bowl, beat ½ cup butter, ¼ cup sugar and the vanilla with an electric mixer until well blended.

On low speed, beat in 1 cup flour until soft dough forms.

Press dough in bottom of pan and bake 10 to 15 minutes or until center is set.

Meanwhile, in 2-quart saucepan, cook filling ingredients over medium-high heat 5 to 10 minutes, stirring frequently, until figs are tender and most of the liquid is absorbed.

Spread over baked crust.

In a small bowl, mix ¼ cup flour, the brown sugar, and 3 tablespoons butter, using pastry blender or fork, until crumbly.

Stir in oats and walnuts. Sprinkle over filling.

Bake 15 to 20 minutes longer or until the edges are bubbly and the top is light golden brown.

Cool completely, about 1 hour.

Cut into bars to serve.

Here is a Second, Different Fig Recipe:

Christopher Wren Gems

Ingredients:

8 oz. dried Calimyrna figs

8 oz. large, dried dates

1 cup plus 1 tbsp Marsala wine

8 oz. cream cheese, room temperature

1/2 cup hazelnuts, toasted and chopped

8 oz. thinly sliced prosciutto

juice of 1/2 lemon

Instructions:

Cut figs in half. Put the figs and dates in a bowl and cover with 1 cup of Marsala and let stand for at least 1 hour.

Process the cream cheese, hazelnuts and 1 tablespoon of Marsala in a food processor until smooth. Refrigerate until cold.

Drain the figs and dates and reserve the Marsala. Slit each date down the center and open the figs to form a pocket. Fill each piece with a teaspoon of the cream cheese mixture.

Preheat oven to 175c/350f.

Close and wrap each piece with a thin strip of prosciutto and sprinkle with reserved marsala.

Place the figs and dates on a baking sheet and bake 7-10 minutes. Let cool and sprinkle with lemon juice.

Fig Bars

Nutrition Facts

Servings: 12

Amount per serving

Calories	**144**

	% Daily Value*
Total Fat 9.4g	**12%**
Saturated Fat 5g	**25%**
Cholesterol 20mg	**7%**
Sodium 55mg	**2%**
Total Carbohydrate 13.6g	**5%**
Dietary Fiber 0.6g	**2%**
Total Sugars 4.3g	
Protein 2g	
Vitamin D 5mcg	27%
Calcium 7mg	1%
Iron 1mg	4%
Potassium 34mg	1%

*The % Daily Value (DV) tells you how much a nutrient in a food serving contributes to a daily diet. 2,000 calorie a day is used for general nutrition advice.

Recipe analyzed

verywell

by

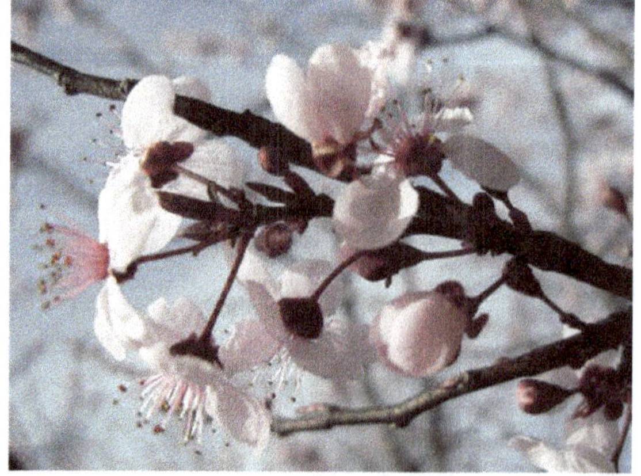

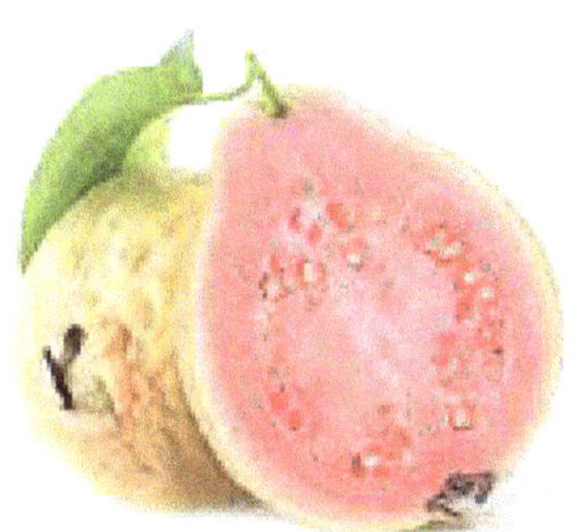

Guava: a fruit that is cultivated and enjoyed in many tropical and subtropical regions. It is a small tree in the Myrtle family, Myrtaceae, native to Mexico, Central America, and northern South America.

Guavas contain four times more fiber than a pineapple and four times more vitamin C than an orange.

Guava is used, in some form or another, to treat an array of ailments including fever, constipation and diarrhea, high blood pressure, hypercholesterolemia and dysentery.

Guava wood is very hard and prized in the world of meat smoking.

In the center of a guava there are between 100-500 edible seeds.

Guavas grow on 20-foot-high evergreen trees, with white flowers.

The leaves of the shrub are a source of black pigment used in textiles.

The lifespan of a plant is 40 years.

The young guava leaves are boiled to make tea to cleanse wounds.

The origin of the guava is unknown, but unofficially the claim is made by Southern Mexico.

There are around 150 varieties of guava.

In El Salvador, the wood of a guava shrub is used to make hair combs.

Columbia has an ancient recipe using guava fruit made into a paste and combined with cheese and eaten with Columbian bread. It is supposedly scrumptious.

Additionally, guava has been attributed to:

-help boost your immunity.

-reduce the risk of developing cancer.

-help manage blood sugar levels.

-help in keeping your heart healthy.

-help during constipation.

-help in improving eyesight.

Guava Recipe:

Guava Bars

Ingredients:

<u>For the crust:</u>

1 cup unsalted butter

1/2 cup sugar

1 tsp salt

2 cups all-purpose flour

<u>For the topping:</u>

16 ounces guava paste, sliced to 1/4-inch thick slices

1 cup old fashioned oats

1/2 cup unsalted butter, diced

1/2 tsp salt

1/2 cup light brown sugar

1 cup all-purpose flour

Instructions:

Grease a 9- by 13-inch baking pan with butter. Adjust oven rack to middle position and preheat oven to 180c/350f.

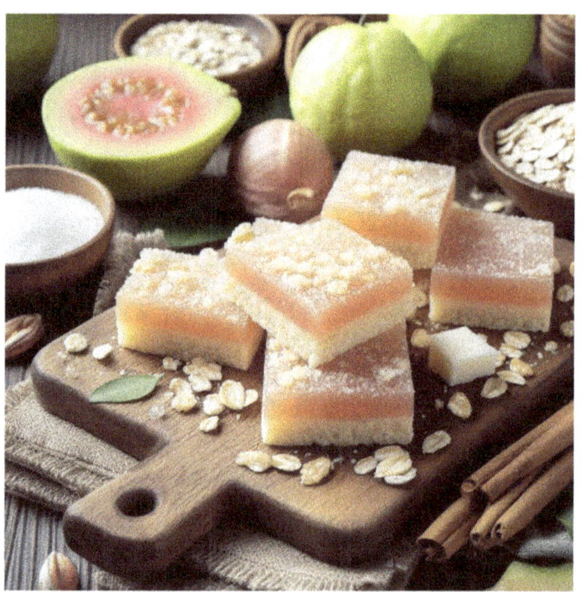

For the crust: Beat butter and sugar together until fluffy, about 3 minutes, then add salt and flour and beat until dough comes together. Press dough evenly into prepared pan. Cover dough with slices of guava paste.

For the topping: Combine oats, butter, salt, and sugar. Pulse 10 times. Add flour and pulse until mixture resembles wet sand. Sprinkle evenly over top of the guava paste. Bake until top is golden, about 45 minutes. Let cool completely before cutting into bars.

Guava Nutritional Facts:

Guava Bars

Nutrition Facts

Servings: 6

Amount per serving

Calories	**589**
	% Daily Value*
Total Fat 32.7g	**42%**
Saturated Fat 19.9g	**99%**
Cholesterol 81mg	**27%**
Sodium 609mg	**26%**
Total Carbohydrate 68.6g	**25%**
Dietary Fiber 6.6g	**24%**
Total Sugars 23.7g	
Protein 8.3g	
Vitamin D 21mcg	106%
Calcium 36mg	3%
Iron 3mg	15%
Potassium 418mg	9%

The % Daily Value (DV) tells you how much a nutrient in a food serving contributes to a daily diet. 2,000 calorie a day is used for general nutrition advice.

Recipe analyzed

verywell

by

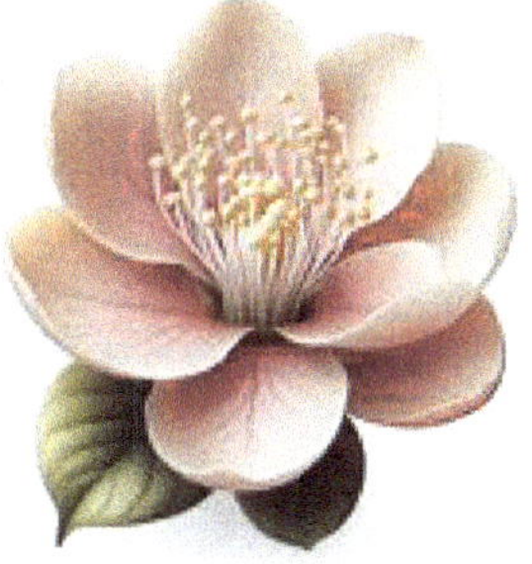

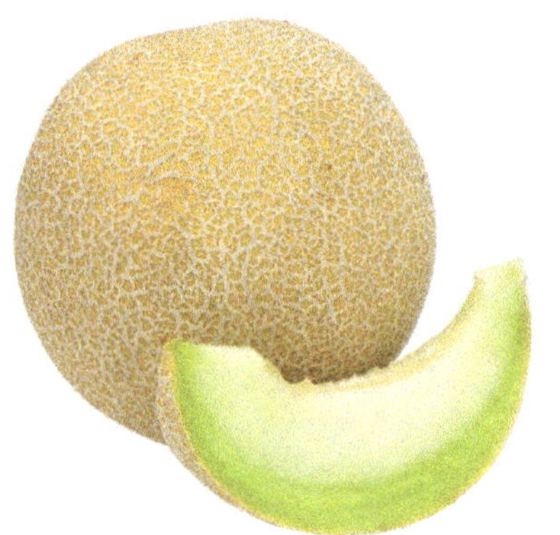

 A melon variety known as honeydew is distinguished by its sweet, juicy flesh and green skin. In addition to antioxidants and fiber, it is a good source of vitamin C and potassium. Fresh honeydew can be consumed as a snack or used in smoothies and fruit salads.

Honeydew melon is a fruit that belongs to the melon species Cucumis melo, along with cantaloupe and other varieties.

Honeydew melon is rich in nutrients, such as folate, vitamin K and magnesium, that may support various aspects of health, such as blood pressure regulation, bone health, digestion and skin health.

Honeydew melon is native to North Africa and southern France, but it is now grown worldwide and available year-round. It can be enjoyed by itself or used in desserts, salads, snacks, and soups.

To choose a ripe honeydew melon, look for one that feels heavy for its size, has a waxy surface and emits a mild, sweet aroma.

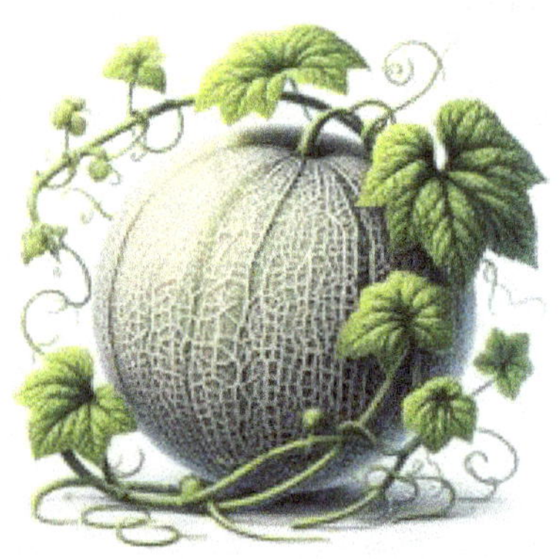

Honeydew Recipe:

Honeydew Melon Agua Fresca with Lime

Ingredients:

1 honeydew melon

1 cup cold coconut water

2 limes

¼ cup honey

Start by picking out a ripe honeydew melon- the color of the rind should be a creamy light-yellow color, not green and the rind should be smooth and waxy. You can also press on the bottom of the honeydew, the opposite end from where it's attached to the vine and give it a little press - it should be slightly soft and springy.

The outside of honeydew melons can hold dirt and other unwanted debris, so make sure to wash the outer rind of the honeydew melon before preparing it.

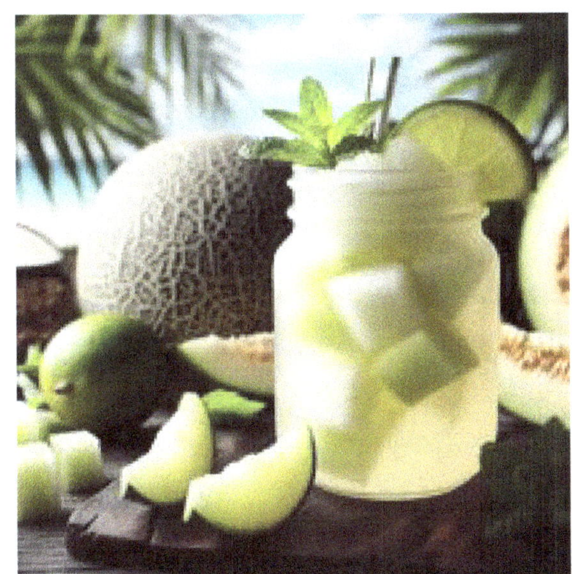

When the honeydew melon has been washed and dried, cut the honeydew melon in half, then remove and discard the seeds with a spoon.

Next, cut the honeydew melon flesh into chunks, make sure to remove the melon from the rind.

Prep the limes by giving them a quick wash, then cut them in half and juice them - if you'd like, juice them directly into a blender, just make sure no lime seeds go into the blender.

Add the honeydew melon chunks, coconut water, fresh lime juice and honey, then blend until the drink is pureed and no chunks remain, about 20-30 seconds.

Strain the mixture through a fine mesh strainer into a large glass pitcher with lid or 64-ounce (2 quart) mason jar, using a wooden spoon to gently press on the pulp to squeeze out the remaining juice, then discard the solids.

Place the drink in the refrigerator to chill for at least 30 minutes or serve immediately over ice. Then enjoy this delicious Honeydew Melon Agua Fresca with lime!

Honeydew Melon Agua Fresca with Lime

Nutrition Facts

Servings: 4

Amount per serving

Calories	**250**

	% Daily Value*
Total Fat 0.3g	**0%**
Saturated Fat 0.1g	**0%**
Cholesterol 0mg	**0%**
Sodium 26mg	**1%**
Total Carbohydrate 68.1g	**25%**
Dietary Fiber 2.5g	**9%**
Total Sugars 62.3g	
Protein 1.2g	
Vitamin D 0mcg	0%
Calcium 28mg	2%
Iron 1mg	4%
Potassium 369mg	8%

*The % Daily Value (DV) tells you how much a nutrient in a food serving contributes to a daily diet. 2,000 calorie a day is used for general nutrition advice.

Recipe analyzed

by **verywell**

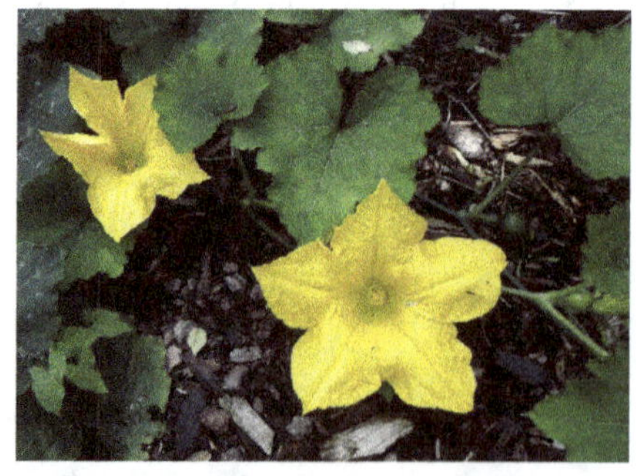

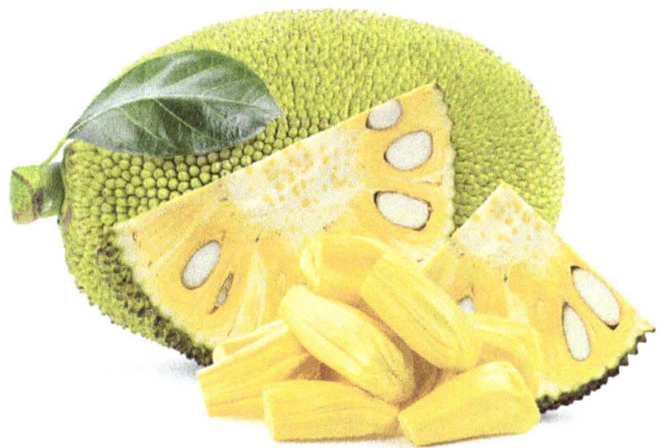

Jackfruit: an exotic fruit grown in tropical regions of the world. It is native to South India and belongs to the same plant family as fig, mulberry and breadfruit. It has a sweet and fruity flavor when ripe and a meat-like texture when unripe. It can weigh up to 40 pounds or more and has a thick, bumpy green rind that covers a stringy yellow flesh.

Jackfruit has a spiky outer skin and is green or yellow in color. One unique aspect of jackfruit is its unusually large size. Jackfruit is the state fruit of the Indian states of Kerala and Tamil Nadu, and it's one of the three auspicious fruits of Tamil Nadu, along with the mango and banana. In Brazil, the jackfruit has become an invasive species as in Brazil's Tijuca Forest National Park in Rio de Janeiro.

Some of the health benefits of jackfruit are:

- It can help lower your blood pressure and prevent heart disease, stroke, and bone loss. This is because it contains potassium, which balances the effects of sodium in your blood vessels.

- It can protect your skin from sun damage and keep it firm and strong. This is because it contains vitamin C, which is an antioxidant that fights free radicals and boosts collagen production.

- It can fight inflammation and promote wound healing. This is because it contains phytochemicals, such as flavonoids, tannins and saponins, which have anti-inflammatory and antibacterial properties.

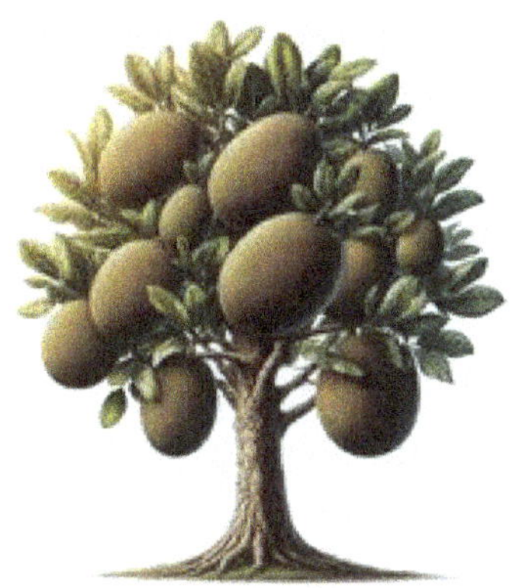

Jack Fruit Recipe:

Annette's Vegan Pulled Pork

Ingredients:

1 jackfruit – not completely ripe, with only a slight aroma

1/2 yellow onion, chopped

4 cloves garlic, minced

3 tsp cumin

3 tsp paprika

2 tsp chili powder

1 tsp black pepper

2 tsp salt

3 tbsps of soy sauce or amino acids

2 tsp mustard

2 cups vegetable broth

1 tbsp olive oil

Prepare the jackfruit:

Cut open the jackfruit and remove pods and stringy "meat". Remove the seeds from the pods and reserve them for another use. This is a messy process as the inside of a jackfruit is very waxy and sticky. Oil your hands and the knife you are using. I like to use a

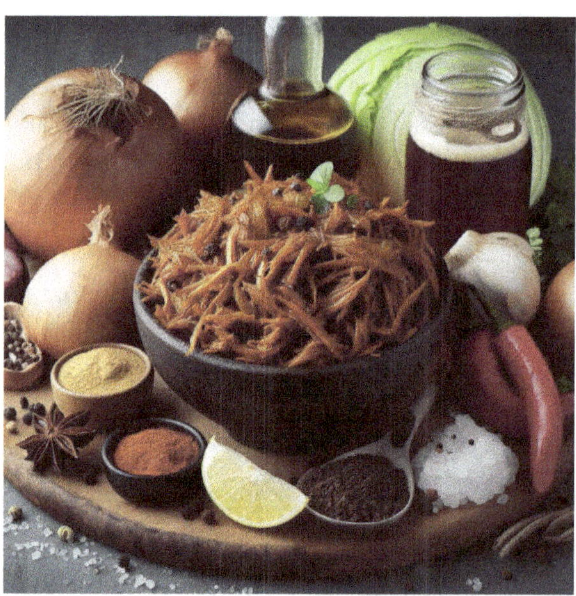

big plastic garbage bag as a surface to keep my counter clean. To clean the knife after, let it

soak in boiling water and the waxy residue will melt off. You can boil and roast the seeds with

salt but that is a separate process.

Recipe follows

Instructions for pulled "pork":

Add oil to large skillet.

Add onions and garlic and cook over medium heat and cook until onions are translucent.

Add jackfruit and all the seasonings to skillet and mix well.

Let simmer for about 5 minutes.

Add veggie stock.

Cover pan and let simmer for 45 minutes.

Preheat oven to 180c/350f

Taste the mixture to see if you would like to add more seasonings (It will taste a little sweet but use your intuition. The baking process will increase the savory flavor.)

Spread the mixture over aluminum foil lined baking sheet.

Place the sheet on the oven's middle rack and cook for 1 hour and 30 minutes.

Enjoy the pulled pork on a sandwich, over rice, over potatoes, or any way you choose.

Annette's Vegan Pulled Pork

Nutrition Facts

Servings: 6

Amount per serving

Calories	**85**
	% Daily Value*
Total Fat 3.7g	**5%**
Saturated Fat 0.6g	**3%**
Cholesterol 0mg	**0%**
Sodium 1493mg	**65%**
Total Carbohydrate 11.2g	**4%**
Dietary Fiber 1.8g	**6%**
Total Sugars 1g	
Protein 3.5g	
Vitamin D 0mcg	0%
Calcium 42mg	3%
Iron 2mg	10%
Potassium 263mg	6%

*The % Daily Value (DV) tells you how much a nutrient in a food serving contributes to a daily diet. 2,000 calorie a day is used for general nutrition advice.

Recipe analyzed

verywell

by

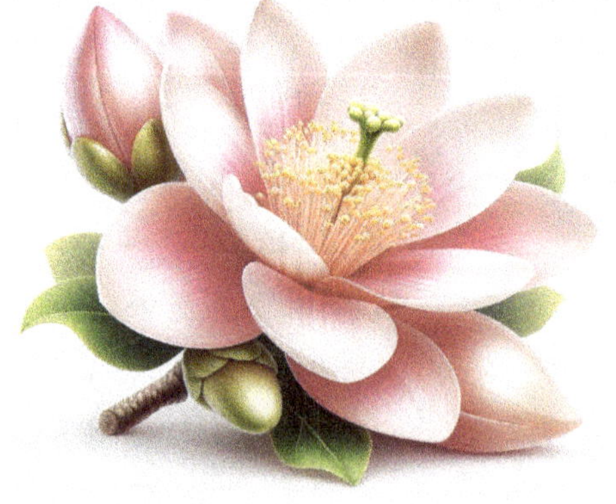

Another way to enjoy jackfruit is to make hummus from its seeds. The seeds are edible and have a nutty flavor. Here is a recipe for **Jackfruit Seed Hummus**:

Ingredients:

2 cups jackfruit seeds

1/4 cup extra virgin olive oil

1/2 cup vegetable broth

1/2 tsp sea salt

3 cloves garlic peeled

1/4 cup garlic spread

1 lemon, juiced

Olive oil and herbs for serving

Instructions:

Clean the jackfruit seeds of any excess membranes from the fruit. Place in a medium saucepan and cover with water until there is at least one inch of water above the seeds. Bring to a boil, then reduce to a simmer and cover. Cook for 30 to 40 minutes, or until seeds can be easily pricked with a fork.

Remove seeds from heat, drain, and cool. Carefully peel off the outer layer of the shell, some of which will have started to pop off during the cooking. Any remaining brown coating on the seed is fine to eat. Add the seeds and all other ingredients to a food processor and puree until smooth. Serve with olive oil, and with herbs of your choice.

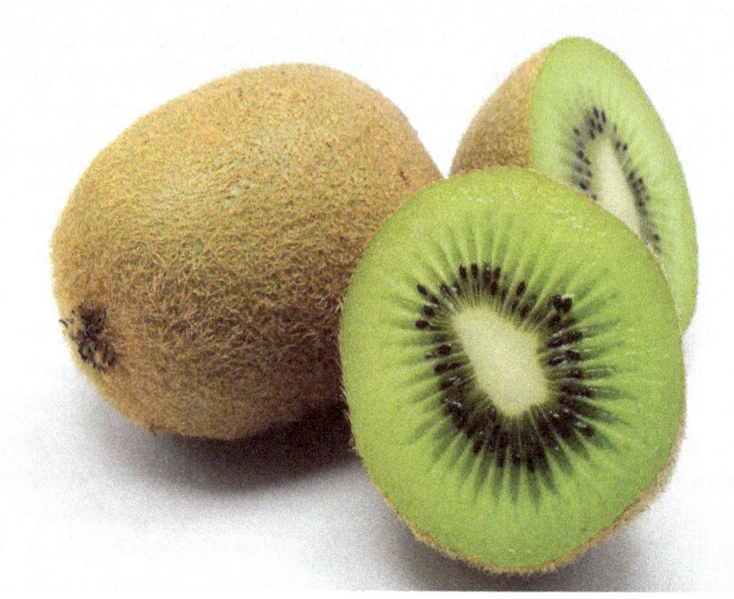

Kiwifruit: A little, tart, sweet fruit originally from China. It has antioxidants, vitamins, and minerals, and is a good source of fiber, potassium, and vitamin C. Kiwifruit can be eaten raw or cooked into desserts, fruit salads, and smoothies.

Kiwifruit is a low-calorie fruit. An average sized kiwifruit, which weighs about 2.7 ounces, has only 46 calories and contains just 0.01 ounces of fat. Kiwi fruits are also incredibly nutritious and loaded with vitamins, folate, and potassium. Unlike many other types of fruit, kiwis have a low glycemic index, which means that they won't cause a strong insulin rush in your body. Did you know that kiwifruits are botanically berries?

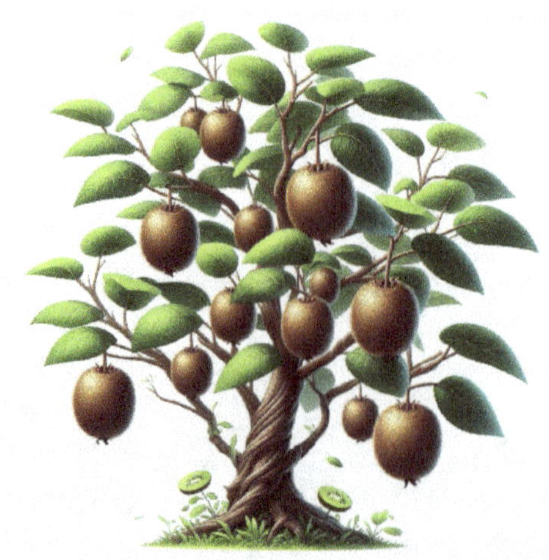

Kiwifruit Quick Bread

Ingredients:

2 cups all-purpose flour

1 tsp baking powder

1⁄4 tsp baking soda

1⁄2 tsp salt

1⁄2 cup butter or margarine (softened)

2⁄3 cup sugar

2 eggs

1 cup peeled mashed kiwifruit

Instructions:

Preheat oven to 180c/350f. Grease and flour a 9 X 5 X 3 loaf pan.

Sift together flour, baking powder, baking soda, and salt and set aside.

In a large bowl cream butter and sugar together until light and fluffy.

Add eggs one at a time, beating well after each one.

Stir in kiwis.

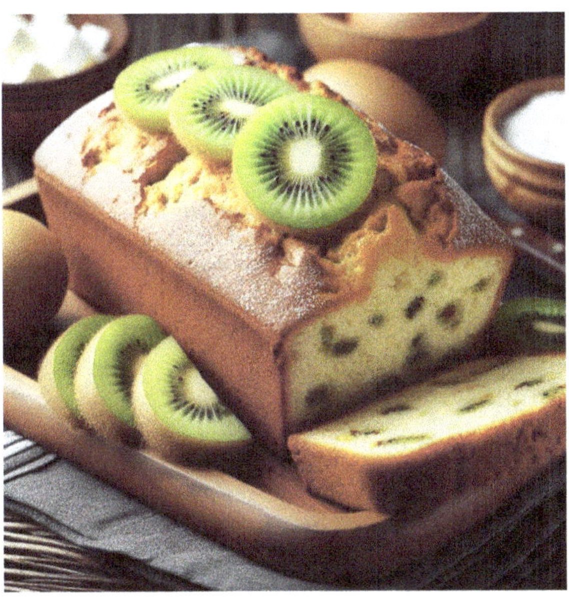

Fold in dry ingredients gently, stirring only until batter is completely moistened.

Spoon batter into a prepared pan and bake for 55-65 minutes or until a toothpick inserted comes out clean.

Cool for 10 minutes on a wire rack. Remove from pan and cool on a rack.

Kiwifruit Quick Bread

Nutrition Facts

Servings: 6

Amount per serving

Calories	**410**

	% Daily Value*
Total Fat 17.4g	**22%**
Saturated Fat 10.2g	**51%**
Cholesterol 95mg	**32%**
Sodium 378mg	**16%**
Total Carbohydrate 58.9g	**21%**
Dietary Fiber 2g	**7%**
Total Sugars 25.1g	
Protein 6.7g	
Vitamin D 16mcg	79%
Calcium 65mg	5%
Iron 2mg	13%
Potassium 245mg	5%

The % Daily Value (DV) tells you how much a nutrient in a food serving contributes to a daily diet. 2,000 calorie a day is used for general nutrition advice.

Recipe analyzed

by **very**well

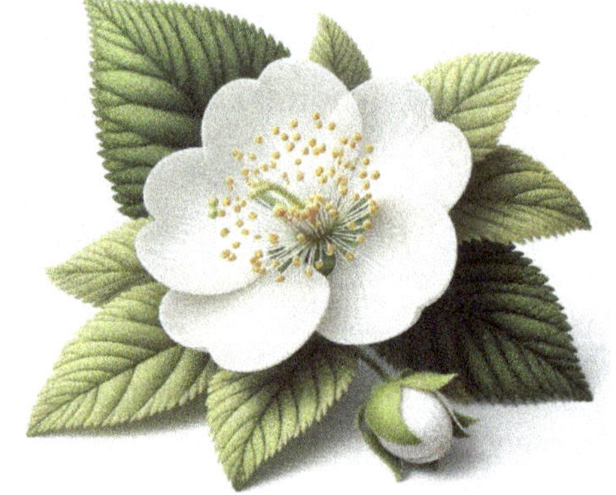

 Citrus fruits, like limes, are popular for their tart flavor and adaptability. They are used as a flavoring agent in foods and beverages as well as in cooking and as a standalone snack.

Limes are sour, round, bright green citrus fruits. They are high in vitamin C, antioxidants, and other nutrients. They may help boost immunity, reduce the chance of heart disease, prevent kidney stones, aid iron absorption, and promote healthy skin.

Did you know that some types of limes are yellow when ripe? The most common lime produced worldwide is the Persian lime (Citrus latifolia), which first became popular and were grown on a large scale in Persia (now Iran).

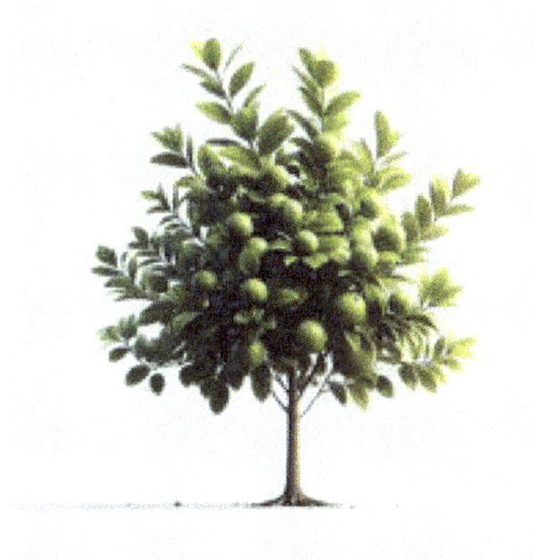

Key Lime Pie

Ingredients:

5 egg yolks, beaten

1 (14 ounce) can sweetened condensed milk

½ cup lime juice

1 (9 inch) graham cracker crust

Instructions:

Preheat the oven to 190c/375f

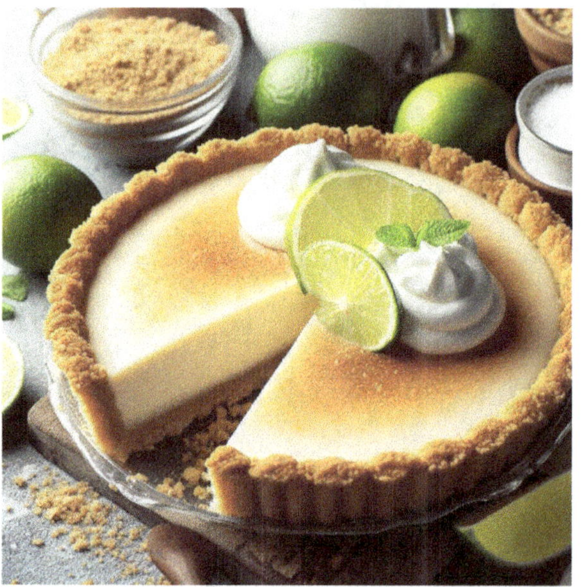

Combine sweetened condensed milk, key lime juice, and egg yolks in a large bowl; mix well

Pour mixture into unbaked graham cracker crust

Bake in the preheated oven until filling is set, about 15 minutes

Allow it to cool completely before slicing

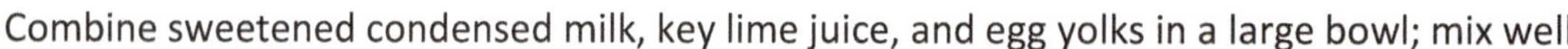

Lime Nutrition Facts:

Key Lime Pie

Nutrition Facts

Servings: 6

Amount per serving

Calories	**481**

	% Daily Value*
Total Fat 20.7g	**27%**
Saturated Fat 7.3g	**37%**
Cholesterol 197mg	**66%**
Sodium 348mg	**15%**
Total Carbohydrate 66.4g	**24%**
Dietary Fiber 0.8g	**3%**
Total Sugars 53.4g	
Protein 9.4g	
Vitamin D 15mcg	76%
Calcium 217mg	17%
Iron 2mg	9%
Potassium 306mg	7%

The % Daily Value (DV) tells you how much a nutrient in a food serving contributes to a daily diet. 2,000 calorie a day is used for general nutrition advice.

Recipe analyzed

verywell

by

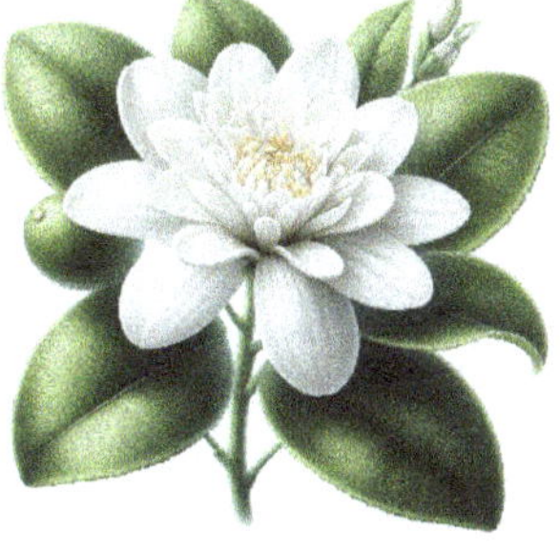

Lychee:

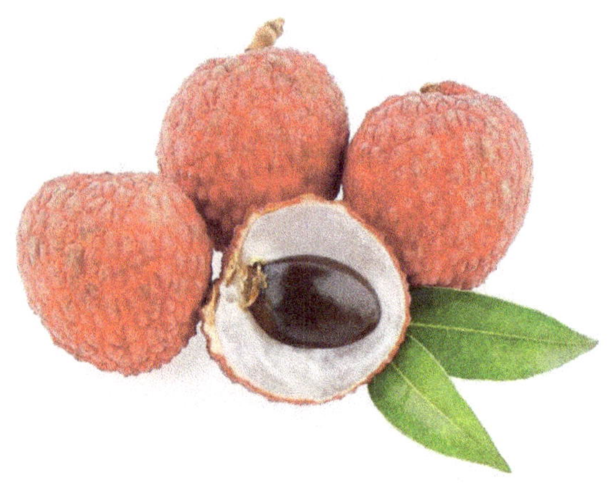

The little, crimson fruit known as lychee is indigenous to China. It tastes slightly flowery and has a sweet, juicy flesh. In addition to potassium and other vitamins and minerals, lychees are a wonderful source of vitamin C, antioxidants, and fiber. They can be consumed raw or used in ice cream, jam, and juice.

Lychee has a floral aroma and a sweet taste that resembles a mix of grape and pear. The flesh has a texture similar to that of a grape. It has been a favorite fruit of the Cantonese since ancient times. It is now grown and enjoyed in the tropics.

Lychee has no saturated fats or cholesterol but comprises good amounts of dietetic fiber, vitamins, and antioxidants. It also has a significant amount of water content, which has a soothing effect on the stomach. Fiber regulates the bowel movement by ensuring its smooth passage through the digestive tract. It also adds bulk to the stool and increases your digestive health.

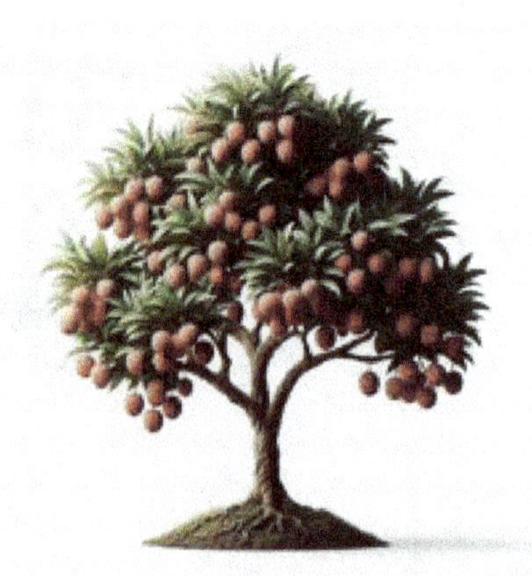

Lychee Recipe:

Refreshing Lychee and Lime Sorbet

Ingredients:

3 cans lychees in syrup

3 tbsp sugar

1 egg white

zest from 2 limes, juice from 1 lime

Instructions:

STEP 1

Drain the syrup from two cans of lychees into a small pan. Add the sugar and dissolve over a gentle heat. Bring to a boil for 1 minute.

STEP 2

Blitz the drained lychees in a food processor until very finely chopped. Pour in the lime juice and syrup with the blade still whirling – don't worry if the mix isn't perfectly smooth at this point. Pour into a 1-litre container and freeze for at least 6 hours until solid.

STEP 3

Break up the frozen mixture, then put it into the bowl of a food processor. Add the egg white and whirl until the mixture is thick, pale, and smooth. Add the zest from 1 lime and whirl again. Return to the container and freeze again, ideally overnight. Serve in scoops with remaining lychees and limes for garnish.

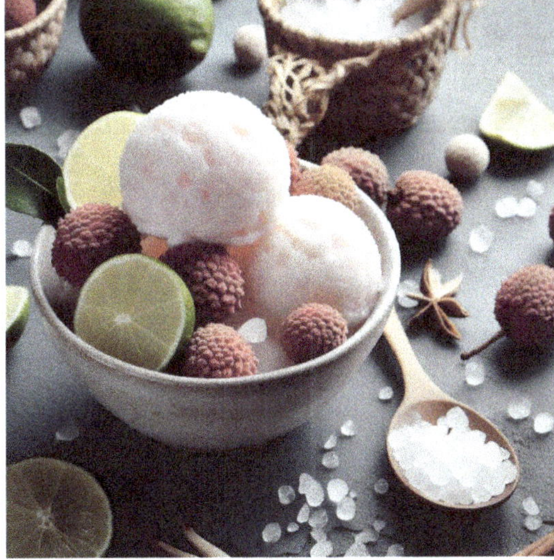

Refreshing Lychee and Lime Sorbet

Nutrition Facts

Servings: 6

Amount per serving

Calories	**44**

	% Daily Value*
Total Fat 0.1g	**0%**
Saturated Fat 0g	**0%**
Cholesterol 0mg	**0%**
Sodium 6mg	**0%**
Total Carbohydrate 11.5g	**4%**
Dietary Fiber 0.7g	**2%**
Total Sugars 9.5g	
Protein 0.8g	
Vitamin D 0mcg	0%
Calcium 8mg	1%
Iron 0mg	1%
Potassium 40mg	1%

The % Daily Value (DV) tells you how much a nutrient in a food serving contributes to a daily diet. 2,000 calorie a day is used for general nutrition advice.

Recipe analyzed

by **very**well

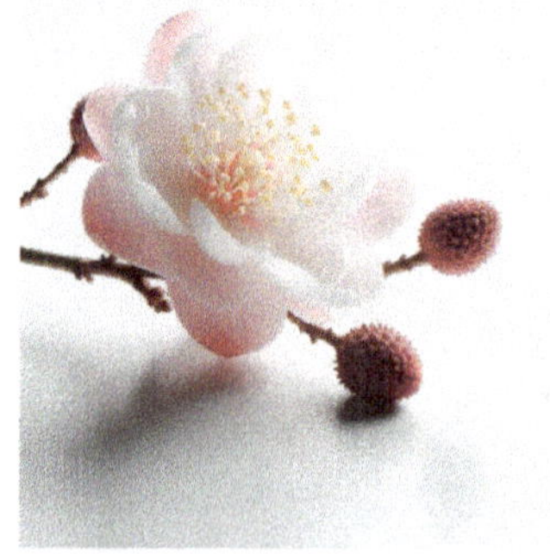

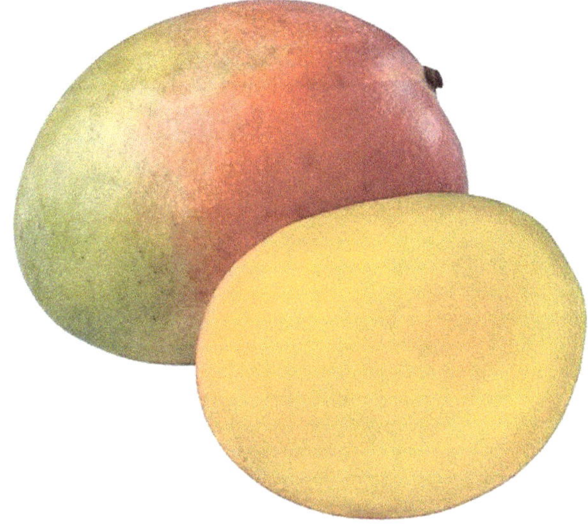

Mango: a tropical fruit that has been treasured for ages. The sweet, juicy, and tasty mango is a fruit that is indigenous to South Asia, and now prolific in Mexico.

It has potassium, vitamins, and minerals, and is a good source of fiber, antioxidants, and vitamin C. Mangoes can be consumed raw, added to juice and smoothies, or used as a foundation for sauces and chutneys.

Mangoes are one of the most popular fruits in the world. They are the succulent, aromatic fruits of an evergreen tree, a member of the cashew family (Anacardiaceous) of flowering plants. Mangoes contain over 20 different vitamins and minerals, most notably vitamin C, vitamin A, folate, fiber, vitamin B6, and copper. One cup (220 grams) of mangoes is just 100 calories, so it's a satisfyingly sweet treat.

Did you know that mango seeds traveled with humans from Asia to the Middle East, East Africa and South America beginning around 300 or 400 A.D.? The species name of the mango is Mangifera indica, which means "an Indian plant bearing mangos."

A basket of mangoes is considered a gesture of friendship in India and the mango is a symbol of love in India. Legend says that Buddha meditated under the cool shade of a mango tree.

In June and July, just before the rainy season, mangoes become ripe, fall from the trees, and flood the streets. There are more mangoes than anyone can eat.

When I walk to the beach, I pick a ripe mango and gorge myself with the sweet juicy nectar. Once at the Mexico beach, I rinse my hands in the salty Pacific Ocean and enjoy the sun and surf. On my way home I cannot resist a second mango, and when I arrive home my hands and mouth are covered in one of nature's most delicious treats.

Mango Recipe:

Mango Chutney

Ingredients:

6 firm but ripe mangoes (about 1.5kg)

2 cups white wine vinegar

3 ½ cups sugar

2 tbsp cumin seeds

2 tsp coriander seeds

10 cardamom pods

½ tsp cayenne pepper

½ tsp turmeric

3 garlic cloves, crushed

8 whole cloves

thumb-sized piece of ginger, grated

1 fat red chile, seeds removed and finely chopped

Instructions:

STEP 1

Peel the mangoes and chop the flesh into blueberry-sized pieces. Pour the vinegar and sugar into a large pan and simmer gently, stirring until the sugar has dissolved. Increase the heat and bubble for 8-10 mins until reduced a little. Meanwhile, toast the cumin, coriander and cardamom in a dry pan until aromatic.

STEP 2

Tip the spices into a mortar and pestle, and gently crush them, leaving the seeds with some texture. Remove the cardamom pods, leaving the seeds in the spice mix, and add to the vinegar mixture along with the mangoes, the other ingredients and 2 tsp salt. Simmer over a medium heat for 1 hr 15 mins – 1 hr 35 mins, until thick and syrupy. Let rest for 10 mins.

STEP 3

Transfer the chutney into 2-3 sterilized jars while still hot. Seal the jars and leave to cool, then add labels. Store in a cool place for up to 2 years – the chutney will be best eaten after a few months, when the flavors have melded and mellowed.

Mango Nutritional Facts:

Mango Chutney

Nutrition Facts

Servings: 6

Amount per serving

Calories	**320**

	% Daily Value*
Total Fat 0.7g	**1%**
Saturated Fat 0.1g	**1%**
Cholesterol 0mg	**0%**
Sodium 12mg	**1%**
Total Carbohydrate 83g	**30%**
Dietary Fiber 1.8g	**6%**
Total Sugars 77.8g	
Protein 1.1g	
Vitamin D 0mcg	0%
Calcium 28mg	2%
Iron 1mg	8%
Potassium 102mg	2%

*The % Daily Value (DV) tells you how much a nutrient in a food serving contributes to a daily diet. 2,000 calorie a day is used for general nutrition advice.

Recipe analyzed

verywell

by

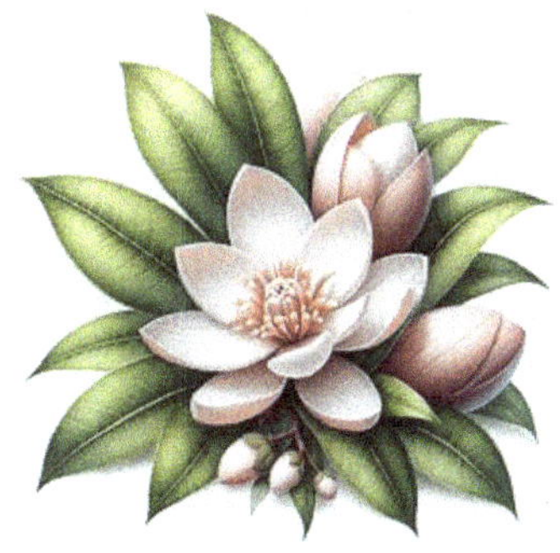

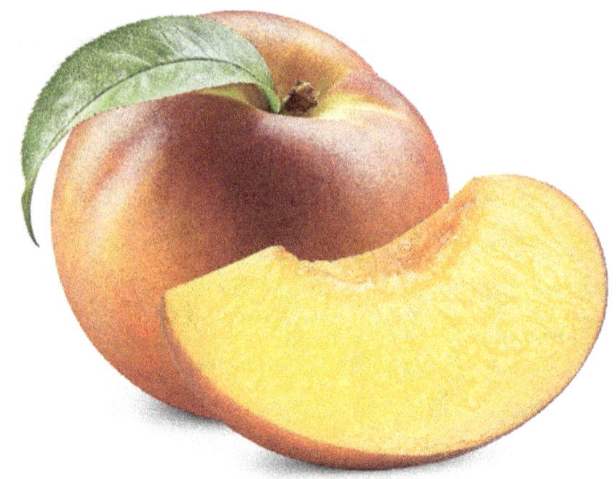

Nectarine: a smooth-skinned stone fruit that is similar to a peach without the fuzz and a slightly different taste. The word nectarine means "sweet as nectar".

Nectarines are low in calories and rich in fiber, vitamin A, vitamin C, and potassium. These nutrients offer health benefits in terms of improved metabolism, digestion, and heart health. You can enjoy nectarines in many ways, such as eating them fresh, adding them to fruit salads, or baking them into delicious desserts. They have yellow or white flesh with a pit in the middle.

Although their flavors are distinct, nectarines and peaches can often be interchanged in recipes.

One medium nectarine, which is approximately 142 grams or 2 1/2 inches in diameter, provides 62 calories. A ripe nectarine is a low-carb fruit that has little fat, some protein, and zero sodium.

Mexico produces almost 165 thousand tons of nectarines each year, which shows the high potential of the Mexican countryside and the people who work it.

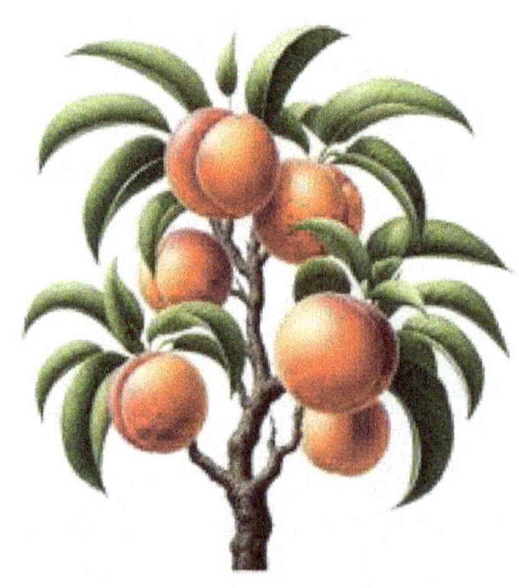

Nectarine Recipe:

Little Nectarine and Cinnamon Picnic Cakes

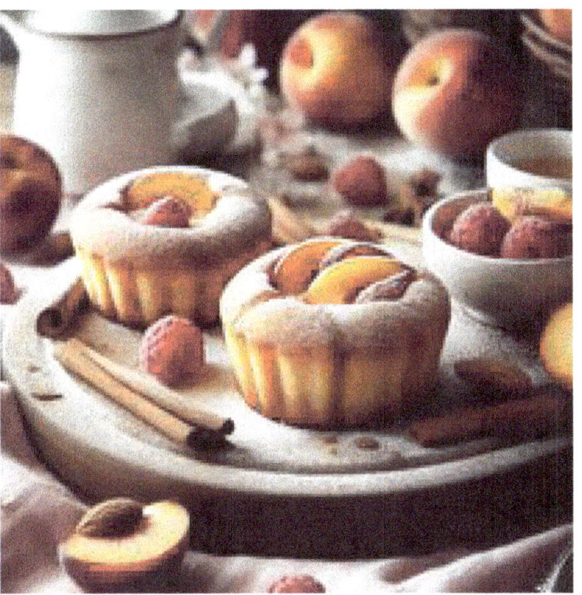

Ingredients:

1 2/3 cups plain flour

3 tbsp ground almonds

2 tsp baking powder

1 tsp ground cinnamon

½ cup soft unsalted butter, chopped

1 cup, firmly packed dark brown sugar

1 tsp vanilla extract

3 eggs, at room temperature

1 cup sour cream

½ cup raspberries

1/3 cup slivered almonds, roasted

3 nectarines, stoned, quartered

Demerara sugar, to sprinkle

Instructions:

Preheat oven to 180°C / 356 F.

Sift flour, almonds, baking powder, cinnamon and 1/2 teaspoon salt into a bowl.

In a separate bowl, using an electric mixer, beat butter, brown sugar, and vanilla until pale and fluffy.

Add eggs one at a time, beating after each.

Add sour cream, beat until just combined, then stir in flour mixture, followed by half the raspberries.

Grease a 6-hole (3/4-cup capacity) muffin tin, scatter slivered almonds among bases, then spoon over batter.

Top each cake with 2 nectarine quarters and scatter with remaining raspberries and a little demerara sugar.

Bake for 35 minutes or until a toothpick inserted into the center comes out clean.

Cool in tins for 5 minutes before turning out.

Little Nectarine and Cinnamon Picnic Cakes

Nutrition Facts	
Servings: 6	
Amount per serving	
Calories	**655**
	% Daily Value*
Total Fat 32.8g	**42%**
Saturated Fat 17.2g	**86%**
Cholesterol 145mg	**48%**
Sodium 186mg	**8%**
Total Carbohydrate 82.6g	**30%**
Dietary Fiber 4.9g	**18%**
Total Sugars 42.9g	
Protein 11.4g	
Vitamin D 19mcg	97%
Calcium 210mg	16%
Iron 3mg	19%
Potassium 593mg	13%

The % Daily Value (DV) tells you how much a nutrient in a food serving contributes to a daily diet. 2,000 calorie a day is used for general nutrition advice.

Recipe analyzed

verywell

by

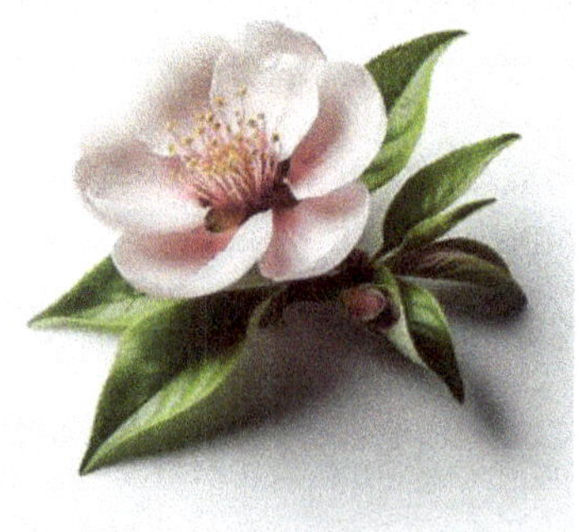

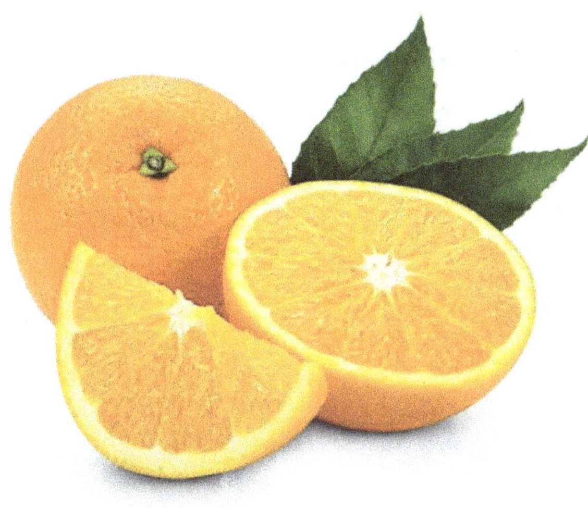

 a citrus fruit that many people like for their sweet and sour taste and juicy flesh. They have a lot of vitamin C and fiber, as well as other nutrients and compounds that can help prevent cancer. Oranges are also rich in flavonoids, which are plant compounds that have anti-inflammatory and antioxidant effects.

You can eat oranges in different ways, such as fresh, as juice, or in salads or jams. Oranges come from a plant called Citrus, which is a hybrid of pomelo and mandarin.

Oranges first grew in a region that includes parts of China, India, and Myanmar, and the Chinese wrote about them in 314 AD. They are now the most common fruit tree in the world. They grow well in warm and sunny places. The aromatic peel is also used in tea and baking

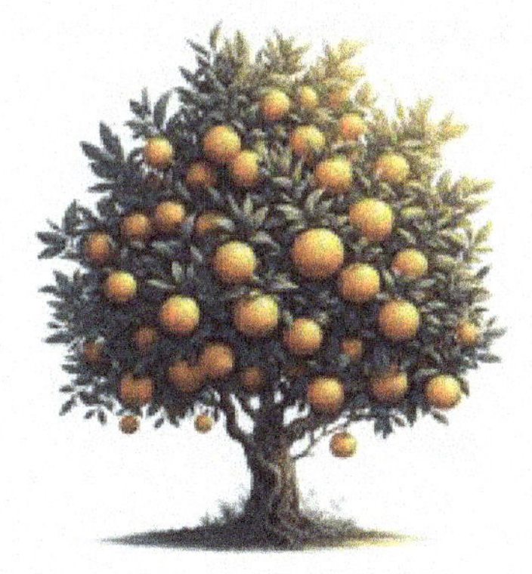

Orange Recipe:

Orange Cheesecake Breakfast Rolls:

Makes 2 dozen

Ingredients:

2 packages (1/4 ounce each) active dry yeast

3/4 cup warm water (110° to 115°)

1-3/4 cups warm 2% milk (110° to 115°)

1 cup sugar

2 large eggs, room temperature

3 tbsp butter, melted

1-1/2 teaspoons salt

7 to 8 cups all-purpose flour

<u>Filling:</u>

1 package (8 ounces) cream cheese, softened

1/2 cup sugar

1 tbsp thawed orange juice concentrate

1/2 tsp vanilla extract

<u>Glaze:</u>

2 cups confectioners' sugar

3 tbsp orange juice

1 tsp grated orange zest

Instructions:

In a large bowl, dissolve yeast in warm water. Then add milk, sugar, eggs, butter, salt and 5 cups flour. Beat until smooth. Stir in enough remaining flour to form a firm dough.

Turn onto a floured surface; knead until smooth and elastic, 6-8 minutes. Place in a greased bowl, turning once to grease the top. Cover and let rise in a warm place until doubled, about 1 hour.

In a small bowl, beat cream cheese, sugar, orange juice concentrate and vanilla until smooth. Punch dough down. Turn onto a lightly floured surface; divide in half. Roll 1 portion into an 18x7 " rectangle. Spread half the filling to within 1/2 " of edges.

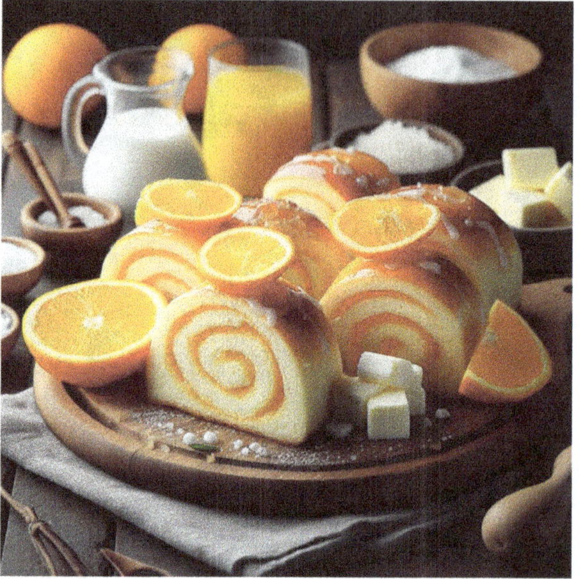

Roll up jelly-roll style, starting with a long side, pinch seam to seal. Cut into 12 slices; place cut side down in a greased 13x9 " baking pan. Repeat with remaining dough and filling. Cover and let rise until doubled, about 30 minutes.

Preheat oven to 175c/350f. Bake rolls for 25-30 minutes or until golden brown. Combine confectioners' sugar, orange juice and zest, drizzle over warm rolls. Refrigerate leftovers.

Orange Cheesecake Breakfast Rolls:

Nutrition Facts

Servings: 12

Amount per serving

Calories 484

	% Daily Value*
Total Fat 7.4g	**9%**
Saturated Fat 4g	**20%**
Cholesterol 48mg	**16%**
Sodium 259mg	**11%**
Total Carbohydrate 94.5g	**34%**
Dietary Fiber 2.3g	**8%**
Total Sugars 37.8g	
Protein 10.3g	
Vitamin D 5mcg	25%
Calcium 48mg	4%
Iron 4mg	21%
Potassium 145mg	3%

*The % Daily Value (DV) tells you how much a nutrient in a food serving contributes to a daily diet. 2,000 calorie a day is used for general nutrition advice.

Recipe analyzed

verywell

by

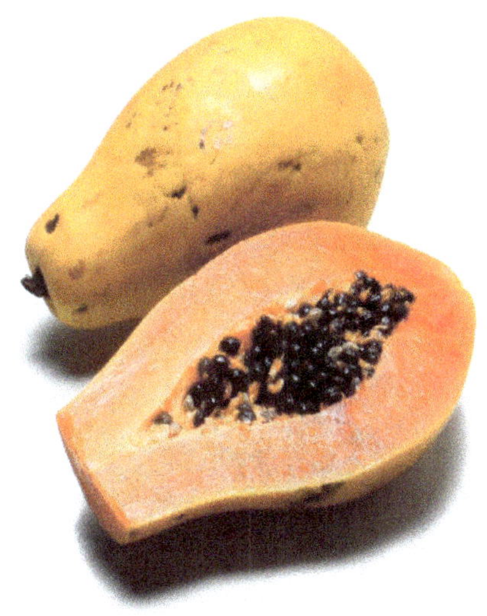

Papaya: a sweet and juicy tropical fruit that comes in orange or pink colors. It has many health benefits, such as vitamin C, folate, potassium, and papain, which aids digestion. The seeds are edible and have a pepper-like flavor.

You can eat papaya fresh, or use it in smoothies, salads, or savory dishes.

The papaya originated in Mesoamerica, where it was first cultivated by the people of southern Mexico and Central America.

Papaya is a small, sparsely branched tree that can grow 10 meters tall. The fruit is a large berry that can be 45 cm long and 30 cm in diameter.

In addition to its nutritional value, papaya has been used for medicinal purposes for centuries. It has been used to treat a variety of ailments, including digestive problems, skin wounds, and infections. Some studies have also suggested that papaya may have anti-inflammatory and antioxidant effects.

Did you know that Christopher Columbus called papaya the "fruit of the angels" when he discovered it in the Caribbean? Papayas are also known by other names around the world. In Australia, and some parts of the United States they are called pawpaws, or papaws, respectively.

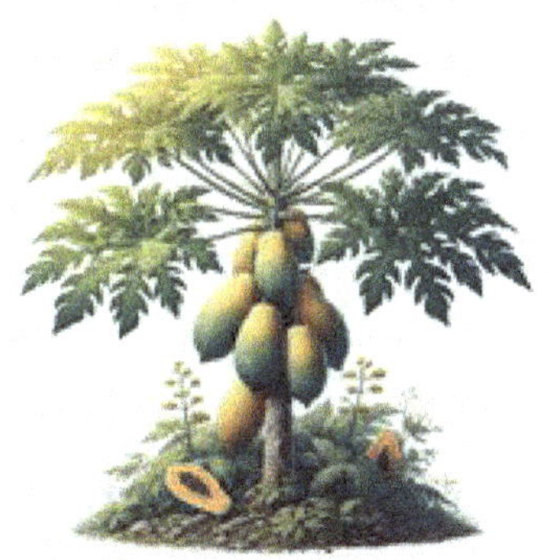

Papaya Recipe:

Mexican Papaya Salad

Ingredients

1/4 cup red onion, thinly sliced

2–3 large handfuls arugula (or other salad greens, or shredded cabbage)

1/2 large ripe papaya, cubed (about 3–4 cups)

1–2 small Turkish cucumbers, sliced

1/4 cup cilantro

1/4 cup toasted coconut

1 tbsp thinly sliced jalapeño

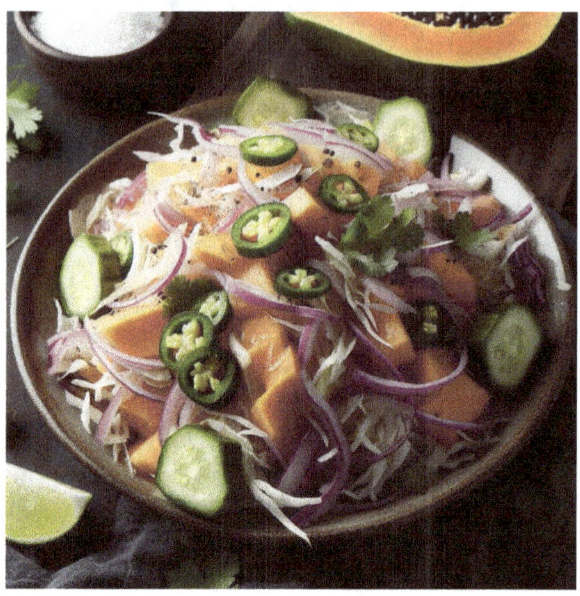

Cilantro Lime Dressing:

Ingredients

3 tbsp olive or avocado oil

1 tbsp lime zest

4 tbsp lime juice

2 tbsp chopped cilantro

1 tbsp chopped scallion

2 tsp honey, agave nectar, or sugar

1/2 tsp coriander

1/4 tsp salt

1/4 tsp pepper

pinch chile flakes or Aleppo

Instructions:

If sensitive to onions, or to remove their "bite", soak thinly sliced onions in salted water while you make the salad. (1/2 teaspoon salt, 1 cup water)

Halve, seed, peel, and cube one half of the papaya, saving the other half for another use. You should have 3-4 cups of 3/4 inch cubes.

Place the greens in a large, wide, serving bowl or on a large platter. Toss with 1/2 of the onions.

Place the papaya on top of the greens.

Slice the cucumber and scatter over the papaya along with remaining onions. At this point, you could refrigerate and serve later that evening.

Make the Cilantro Lime Dressing by mixing all ingredients together in a small bowl or jar. Spoon it over the salad right before serving, tossing gently.

Sprinkle with cilantro leaves, optional jalapeño and toasted coconut.

Add more lime to taste.

Papaya Nutritional Facts:

Mexican Papaya Salad

Nutrition Facts

Servings: 4

Amount per serving

Calories	**168**

	% Daily Value*
Total Fat 12.5g	**16%**
Saturated Fat 3g	**15%**
Cholesterol 0mg	**0%**
Sodium 157mg	**7%**
Total Carbohydrate 16.8g	**6%**
Dietary Fiber 2.4g	**9%**
Total Sugars 9.6g	
Protein 1.4g	
Vitamin D 0mcg	0%
Calcium 39mg	3%
Iron 1mg	7%
Potassium 310mg	7%

*The % Daily Value (DV) tells you how much a nutrient in a food serving contributes to a daily diet. 2,000 calorie a day is used for general nutrition advice.

Recipe analyzed

verywell

by

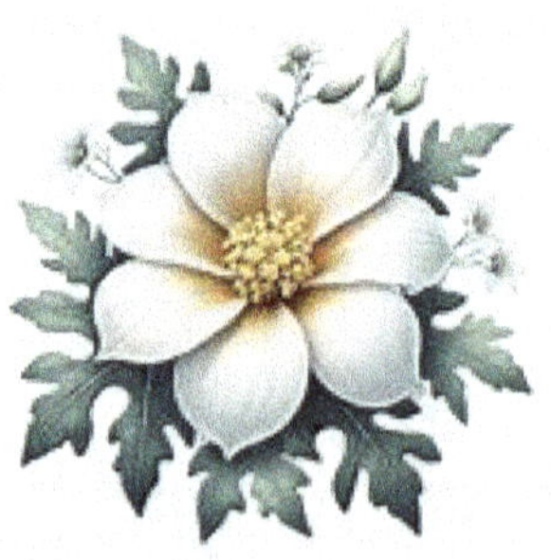

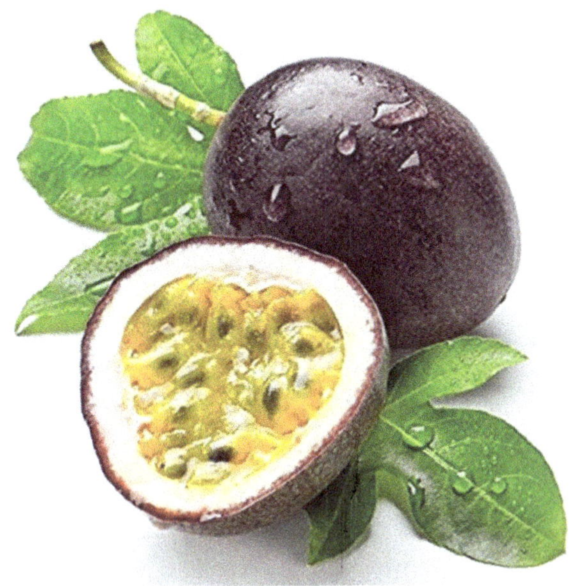

 a small and round fruit that can be purple or yellow. It has a sweet and sour flavor, and it is a good source of fiber, vitamin C, and antioxidants.

You can eat it fresh, use it in desserts, or make juices and smoothies with it. The passion fruit plant (Passiflora edulis) belongs to the Passifloraceae family and has two main varieties: the purple passion fruit and the yellow passion fruit. It is a woody evergreen vine that grows fast and climbs with tendrils. It has glossy leaves with three lobes and serrated edges that are arranged alternately. It produces fruit about 80 days after flowering in the warmest months of the year (summer to fall). The roots of the vine are shallow, and the stem is woody.

The fruit of both varieties is climacteric, meaning it ripens after being picked. It also produces a lot of ethylene gas.

The purple passion fruit has a dark-purple or almost black skin and is round or oval. It is about 5 cm long and weighs 30-45 g.

The yellow passion fruit has a deep yellow skin that is similar in shape but slightly longer (6 cm) and bigger than the purple one. It weighs 60-90 g and averages about 75 g.

The fruit has a thick rind with a white pith inside. The pith surrounds a cavity that contains up to 250 small black seeds. Each seed is covered by an orange sac that holds the juicy pulp, which is the edible part of the fruit. The pulp has a musky and guava-like aroma and a slightly acidic taste.

Passion fruit has very distinctive and beautiful flowers that make it a popular ornamental plant. The flowers look like clocks, have white and purple-blue colors (especially in the center), five petals, three large green bracts, and a diameter of about 4.5-6 cm, depending on the variety of passion fruit. The flower also has five stamens with big anthers, an ovary, and a three-branched style that forms a striking central structure.

Pollination is vital for fruit production on passion vines. Purple passion vines can self-pollinate and produce fruit, but yellow passion vines need cross-pollination from another compatible vine. Passion vines need mild temperatures to fruit well and may not produce usable fruit during the hottest part of the hot season. Bees are the most effective insects for pollinating passion fruit flowers.

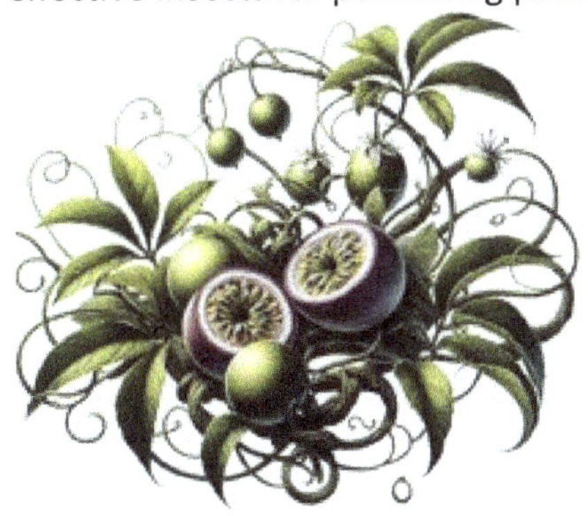

Passion Fruit Recipe:

Passion Fruit Scones

Ingredients:

3 cups self-rising flour, plus extra to dust

1/3 cup cold butter

1 tbsp caster sugar

1 cup white chocolate

1 cup milk, plus extra to brush

1/3 cup fresh passionfruit pulp

Whipped cream, to serve

STEP 1

Preheat oven to 200c/380f fan forced. Line an

oven tray with parchment paper.

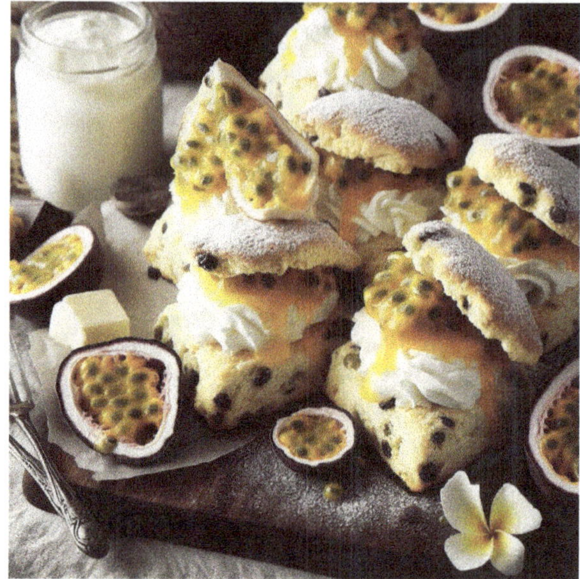

STEP 2

Place the flour in a large bowl. Add the butter and use your fingertips to rub the butter into the flour until it resembles fine breadcrumbs. Stir in sugar and chocolate.

STEP 3

Make a well in the center. Pour the milk and passionfruit pulp into the well. Use a non-serrated knife to mix until it starts to form clumps of dough and there is no dry flour.

STEP 4

Turn dough onto a lightly floured surface and gather together. Gently press out to shape dough into a ¾" / 2cm thick disc. Use a floured 2" / 6cm round cutter to cut out 16 scones, dipping the cutter in extra flour between cuts. Arrange scones, just touching, on the prepared tray. Brush tops lightly with extra milk.

STEP 5

Bake for 15 minutes or until risen and golden brown. Slide onto a wire rack and cool slightly. Serve warm or at room temperature, with whipped cream.

Passion Fruit Nutritional Facts:

Passion Fruit Scones

Nutrition Facts

Servings: 6

Amount per serving

Calories	**3394**

	% Daily Value*
Total Fat 205.6g	**264%**
Saturated Fat 131.5g	**658%**
Cholesterol 54mg	**18%**
Sodium 650mg	**28%**
Total Carbohydrate 374.4g	**136%**
Dietary Fiber 2.1g	**7%**
Total Sugars 228.5g	
Protein 18.2g	
Vitamin D 6mcg	29%
Calcium 138mg	11%
Iron 4mg	20%
Potassium 213mg	5%

**The % Daily Value (DV) tells you how much a nutrient in a food serving contributes to a daily diet. 2,000 calorie a day is used for general nutrition advice.*

Recipe analyzed

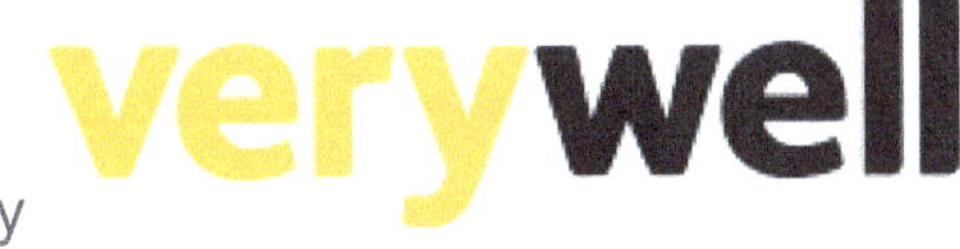

by

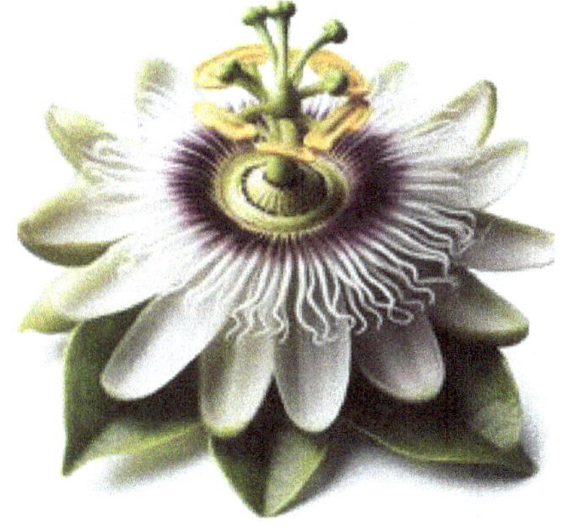

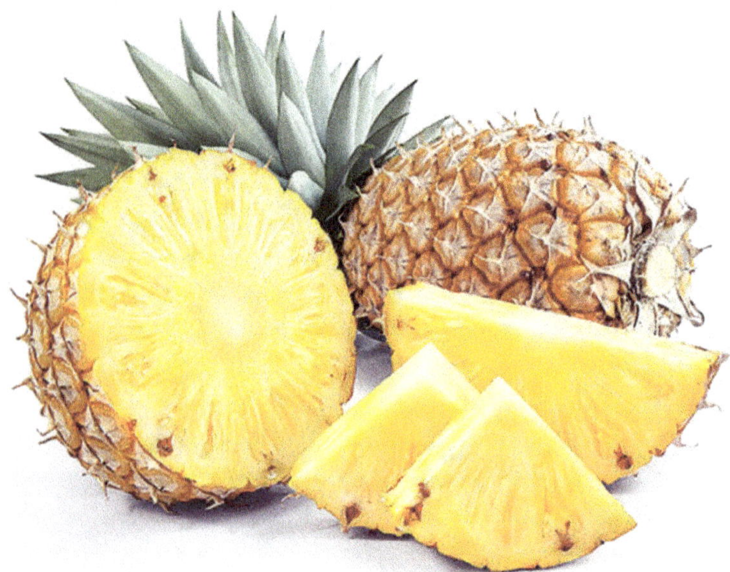

Pineapple: a tropical fruit that originated in South America. It has a sweet and slightly sour flavor and is rich in vitamin C, fiber, antioxidants, and bromelain, an enzyme that can help with digestion and inflammation.

You can enjoy pineapples in various ways, such as eating them fresh, making smoothies or salsa with them, or adding them to your dishes.
The pineapple (Ananas comosus) is a plant that belongs to the Bromeliaceous family. It is the most important plant in this family in terms of economic value.

The pineapple has been grown in South America for a long time.
There are several ways to select a ripe pineapple:

1. Look for a pineapple that has a greenish-yellow color, especially around the spiny points. Avoid pineapples that are mostly green or deep yellow to orange, as they may be underripe or overripe respectively.
2. Squeeze the pineapple gently and feel for a firm but slightly soft texture. Pineapples that are too hard or too soft may not be ripe.
3. Smell the base of the pineapple and check for a sweet aroma. If the pineapple has no smell or a pungent or bitter smell, it may not be ripe or may be spoiled.
4. Pick a pineapple that feels heavy for its size, which means it is juicier and sweeter.
5. Pull on the fronds (the large leaves on top of the pineapple) and see if they come out quickly. This may indicate that the pineapple is ripe and ready to eat.
6. Choose a pineapple with bigger eyes (the diamond-shaped patterns on the skin), which means it was left to ripen longer before being picked. Also, look for a pineapple with a plump, round body instead of one that tapers too much at the top.

Pineapple Recipe:

Pineapple Meringue Pie

Ingredients:

For the meringues:

3 egg whites
½ cup caster sugar
2 tsp corn flour
1 tsp lemon juice

For the cream:

1 cup crème fraiche
1/8 cup icing sugar
¼ tsp vanilla extract

For the fruit salad:

1 cup pineapple, chopped into small chunks
2 passion fruit, pulp scooped out
mint leaves, shredded (optional)

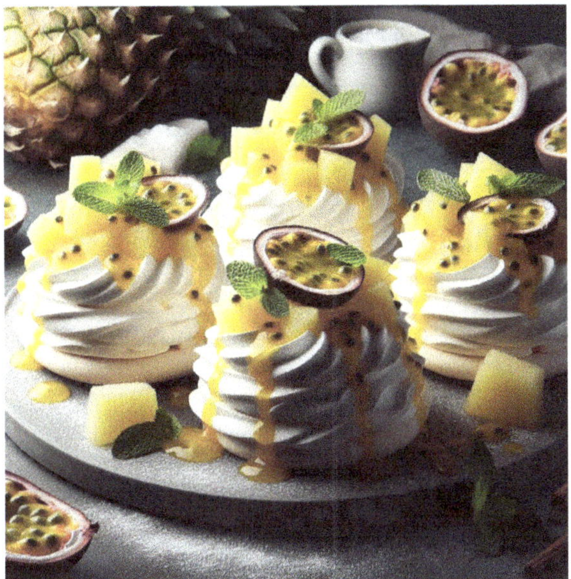

STEP 1

Heat the oven to 120c/250f fan/gas 1. Line a baking sheet with parchment paper. Draw four circles, 3" / 8cm in diameter, on the baking parchment, then flip over. Whisk the egg whites in a large bowl using an electric whisk until stiff peaks form. Gradually whisk in the sugar until thick and glossy, then the corn flour and lemon juice. Pile the meringue in swirls onto the marked circles, making a dip in the middle, then bake on the lowest shelf for 55 mins-1 hr until crisp on the outside and dry underneath. Turn the oven off, leave the oven door ajar and leave the meringue to cool completely. These can be made a day ahead and kept in an airtight container.

STEP 2

Whisk the crème fraiche in a bowl with the icing sugar and vanilla extract until thick and pillowy. Mix the pineapple and passion fruit together in a separate bowl. To assemble, spoon a quarter of the crème fraiche mixture onto each meringue, top with pineapple and passion fruit mixture. Finish with mint leaves to serve if you like.

Pineapple Nutritional Facts:

Pineapple Meringue Pie

Nutrition Facts

Servings: 4

Amount per serving

Calories 185

	% Daily Value*
Total Fat 0.3g	0%
Saturated Fat 0g	0%
Cholesterol 0mg	0%
Sodium 29mg	1%
Total Carbohydrate 45.1g	16%
Dietary Fiber 1.9g	7%
Total Sugars 41.1g	
Protein 3.4g	
Vitamin D 0mcg	0%
Calcium 15mg	1%
Iron 1mg	4%
Potassium 145mg	3%

*The % Daily Value (DV) tells you how much a nutrient in a food serving contributes to a daily diet. 2,000 calorie a day is used for general nutrition advice.

Recipe analyzed

verywell

by

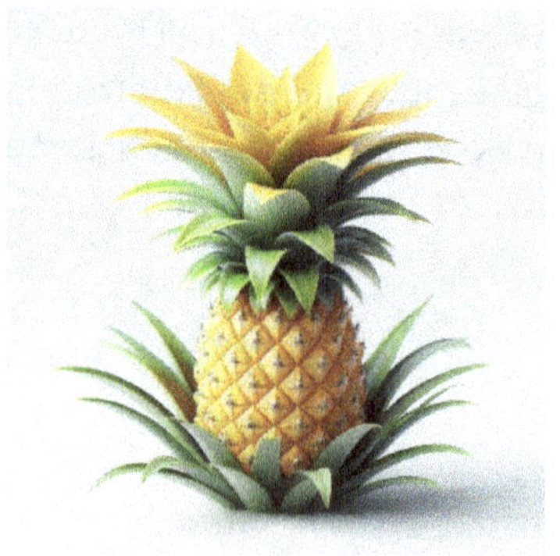

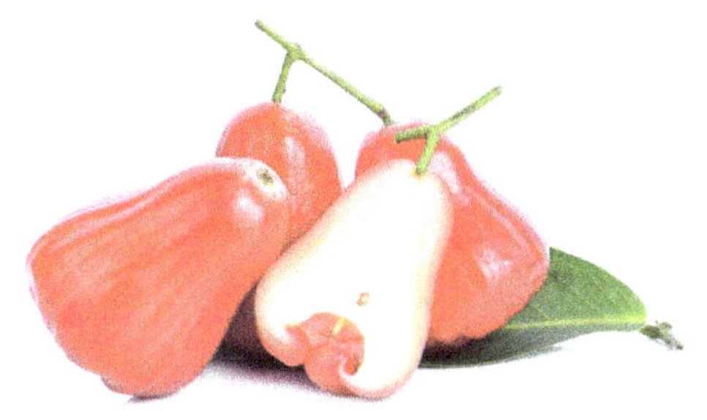

<u>Pomarosa:</u> (*Syzygium jambos*) is a fruit originating in Southeast Asia and now found in various other regions where it has been introduced as an ornamental and fruit tree.

 Pomarosa is a large shrub or small-to-medium-sized tree, typically 3 to 15 meters (10 to 49 feet) high. Its leaves are lanceolate, 2 to 4 centimeters broad and 10 to 20 centimeters long. The flowers are in small terminal clusters, white or greenish white, with numerous stamens. The fruit resembles some types of guavas but has distinct fragrance, flavor, and texture. Instead of many small, hard seeds, it usually contains one or two large, unarmored seeds about a centimeter in diameter. The skin is thin and waxy, and the ripe fruit has a strong, pleasant floral bouquet, which is why it's also known as "rose apple" or "pomarosa".

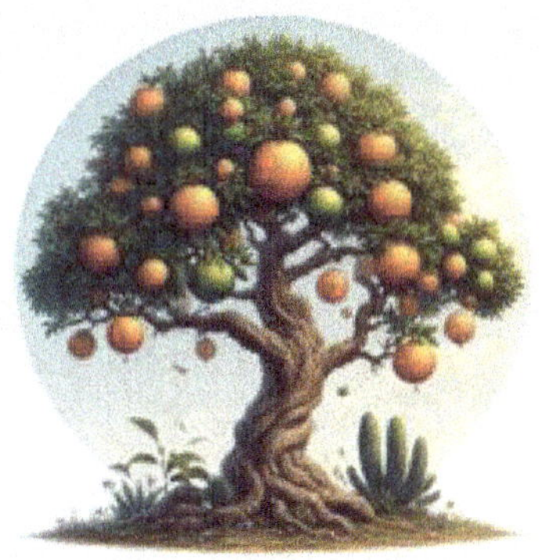

Pomarosa Recipe:

Dulce de Pomarosa

Ingredients:

5 pomarosas

1 cup of sugar

1 cinnamon stick

1 tbsp vanilla extract

Instructions:

Slice each pomarosa in half and remove the seeds

Place the pomarosa halves in a Mexican clay pot

Sprinkle the sugar over the pomarosas.

Add the cinnamon stick and vanilla extract to the clay pot.

Bring the mixture to a boil over medium heat

Once it starts boiling, reduce the heat to low

Let it simmer for about 30-40 minutes, until the pomarosas are tender and the syrup has thickened

Cool and serve

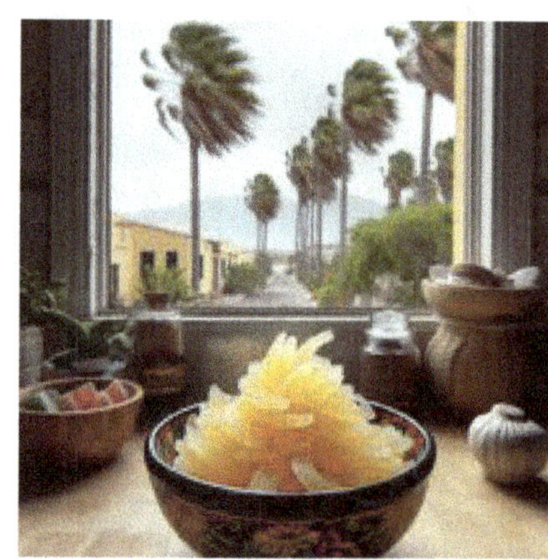

Pomarosa Nutritional Facts:

Dulce de Pomarosa

Nutrition Facts

Servings: 6

Amount per serving

Calories	163

	% Daily Value*
Total Fat 0.4g	0%
Saturated Fat 0.1g	1%
Cholesterol 0mg	0%
Sodium 4mg	0%
Total Carbohydrate 34.6g	13%
Dietary Fiber 9.8g	35%
Total Sugars 20.6g	
Protein 1.1g	
Vitamin D 0mcg	0%
Calcium 172mg	13%
Iron 1mg	8%
Potassium 166mg	4%

*The % Daily Value (DV) tells you how much a nutrient in a food serving contributes to a daily diet. 2,000 calorie a day is used for general nutrition advice.

Recipe analyzed

verywell

by

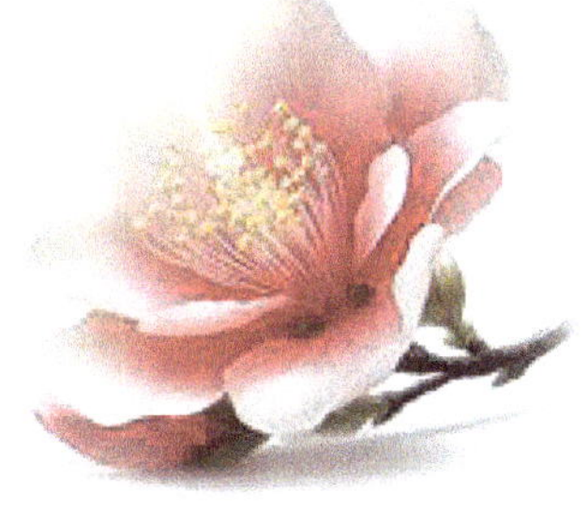

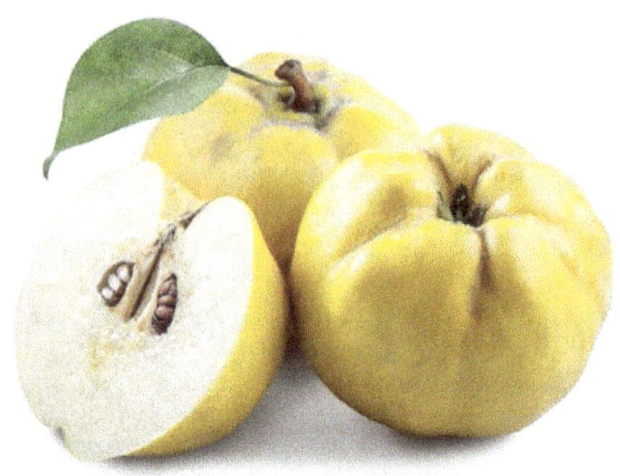

Quince: a hard, yellow fruit that belongs to the same family as apples and pears. It has a unique flavor that is both sweet and sour, and it is often cooked or baked to make jams, pies, and other delicacies.

Quince is rich in fiber, vitamins, and minerals, such as potassium and vitamin C. The quince (Cydonia oblonga) is the only species in the Cydonia genus of the Rosaceae family. It grows on a deciduous tree that produces bright golden-yellow pome fruits that resemble pears.

Quince fruits are hard, sour, and fragrant when ripe. They are rarely eaten raw, but are used to make marmalade, jam, paste (also called quince cheese) or alcoholic drinks.

The flowers bloom 2+1/2–4+1/2 " in spring after the leaves emerge, and are white or pink, with five petals.

The young fruit is green and covered with fine white hairs that mostly fall off by late autumn when the fruit turns yellow, and the flesh becomes firm and aromatic. The leaves are simple, alternately arranged, 60–110 mm long, with smooth edges and fine white hairs on both sides.

Quince has been used in folk medicine for decades, but scientific research on its benefits is still in the early stages.

Quinces contain fiber and several essential vitamins and minerals, making them a nutritious addition to almost any diet.

Quinces offer a rich supply of antioxidants, which may reduce metabolic stress and inflammation while protecting your cells from free radical damage.

Quince syrup has been found to be significantly more effective than vitamin B6 at reducing pregnancy-induced nausea and vomiting.

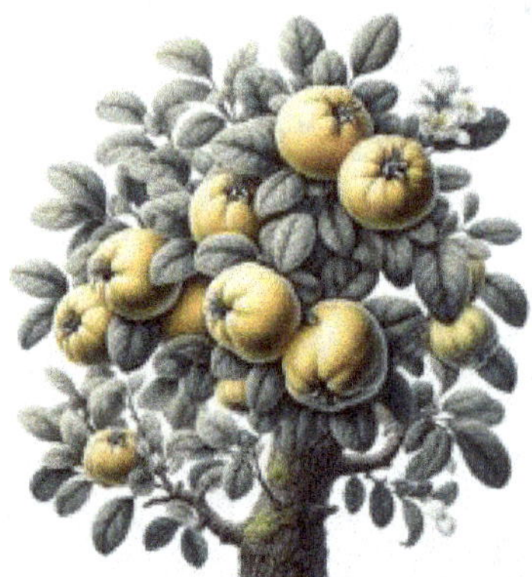

Quince Recipe:

Baked Quince

Ingredients:

4 quinces, peeled, cored, and cut in half

1/2 cup unsalted butter, divided

1 cup sugar, divided

1 cup hot water

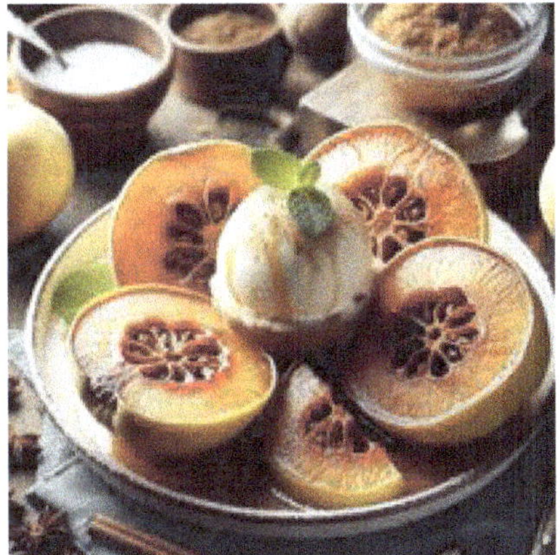

Instructions:

Preheat oven to 350 F.

Place the quince halves in a 9-by-12-inch baking dish, cut-side up. Top each quince half with 1 tbsp of butter and sprinkle with 2 tbsp of sugar. Pour the hot water around the quince halves without disturbing the topping.

Bake in the preheated oven until the quinces are a golden color and soft, about 1 to 1 1/2 hours.

Remove the baking dish to a rack and let stand for 15 minutes before serving.

Serve with ice cream, whipped cream, custard sauce, or with cooking liquids.

Tips:

To keep the quince halves from browning as you prepare them, brush with lemon juice.

A pitting spoon is handy for removing the tough cores. Or try using an apple corer, peach pitter, or melon baller.

Recipe Variations:

Replace all or part of the water with apple juice or apple cider.

For a warm spice flavor, combine the sugar with 2 to 3 tbsp of ground cinnamon.

For caramel flavor, replace the granulated sugar with brown sugar.

How to Store Baked Quinces:

Refrigerate baked quince halves with the juices in an airtight container for up to 5 days.

Quince Nutritional Facts:

Baked Quince

Nutrition Facts

Servings: 8

Amount per serving

Calories	**222**

	% Daily Value*
Total Fat 11.6g	15%
Saturated Fat 7.3g	36%
Cholesterol 31mg	10%
Sodium 84mg	4%
Total Carbohydrate 32.1g	12%
Dietary Fiber 0.9g	3%
Total Sugars 25g	
Protein 0.3g	
Vitamin D 8mcg	40%
Calcium 9mg	1%
Iron 0mg	2%
Potassium 94mg	2%

*The % Daily Value (DV) tells you how much a nutrient in a food serving contributes to a daily diet. 2,000 calorie a day is used for general nutrition advice.

Recipe analyzed

verywell

by

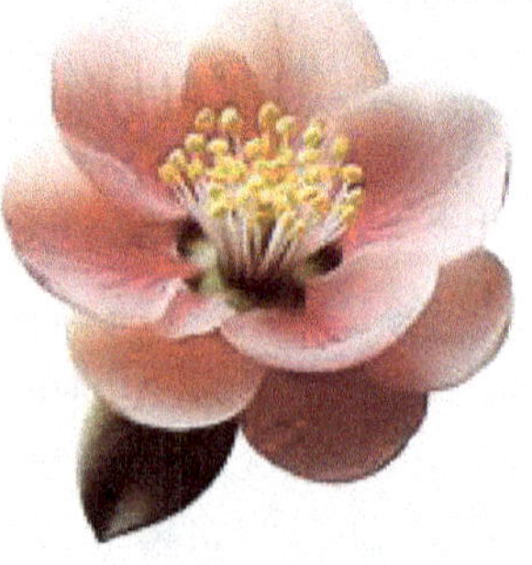

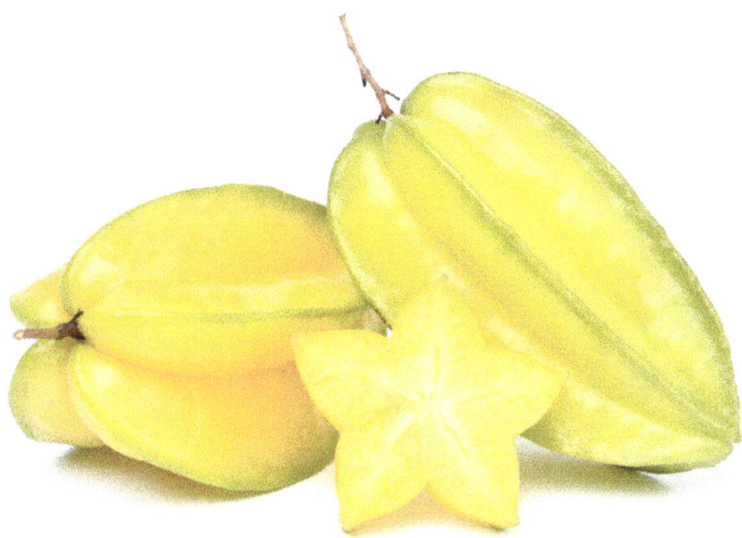

Star fruit: is a tropical fruit that grows on Averrhoa carambola trees in Southeast Asia and Mexico.

 It has a yellow color and a star shape when sliced. The fruit tastes sweet and sour and can be used in various dishes and drinks.

It is also rich in vitamin C, fiber, and antioxidants, which are beneficial for your health.

Star fruit has a high oxalate content, which is not good for kidneys. They are also extremely toxic to dogs.

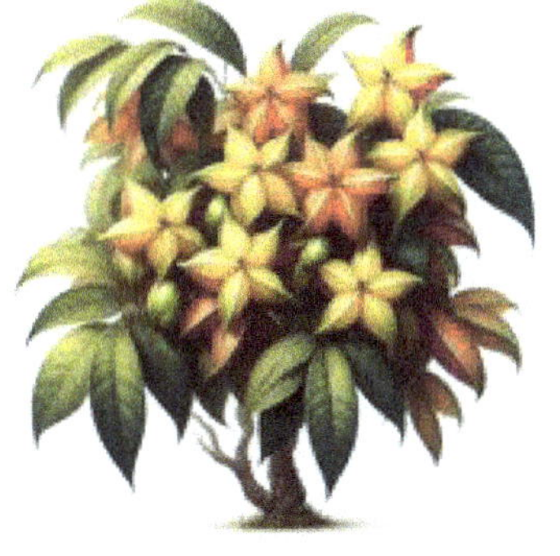

Star fruit Recipe:

Star Fruit Chip

Easy star fruit chips in a pumpkin spice for a low carb sweet snack

Ingredients:

2 star fruits

2 tbs pumpkin spice

Instructions:

Preheat the oven to 200C/400F.

Thinly slice the star fruits.

Gently remove the seeds with a teaspoon.

Place the slices in a bowl and sprinkle the pumpkin spice over them. Mix well to ensure that all slices are covered.

Place the slices on a parchment lined baking tray.

Bake for 30-35 until crisp (flip over halfway through cooking time). Ovens can vary so you may need more time.

Star Fruit Chip

Nutrition Facts

Servings: 8

Amount per serving

Calories	**93**

	% Daily Value*
Total Fat 3.2g	4%
Saturated Fat 1.6g	8%
Cholesterol 0mg	0%
Sodium 14mg	1%
Total Carbohydrate 19g	7%
Dietary Fiber 4.4g	**16%**
Total Sugars 2.9g	
Protein 1.7g	
Vitamin D 0mcg	0%
Calcium 171mg	13%
Iron 5mg	28%
Potassium 199mg	4%

*The % Daily Value (DV) tells you how much a nutrient in a food serving contributes to a daily diet. 2,000 calorie a day is used for general nutrition advice.

Recipe analyzed

by **verywell**

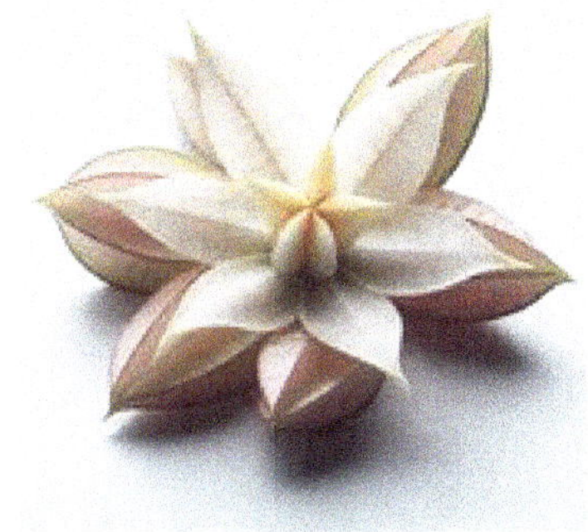

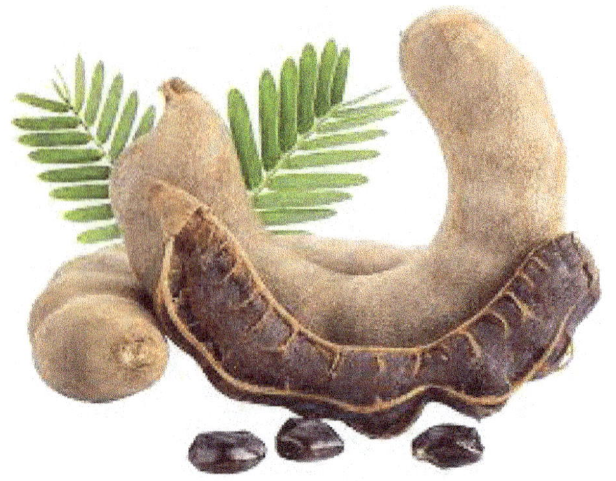

Tamarind: A sour and tangy pulp inside a brown pod is the fruit of the tamarind tree, which is often used to add flavor to various dishes and beverages in Mexico and Southeast Asian cuisine.

Tamarind provides many health benefits as it is rich in vitamin B6, potassium, and other antioxidants and anti-inflammatory substances.

Tamarind is the only species in its genus, and it belongs to the legume family. It is native to tropical Africa and has spread to Asia and Mexico.

It is used in traditional medicine to treat various ailments such as constipation, fever, and inflammation.

Tamarind contains high levels of tartaric acid, which gives it its sour taste. Tartaric acid is also found in wine and grapes.

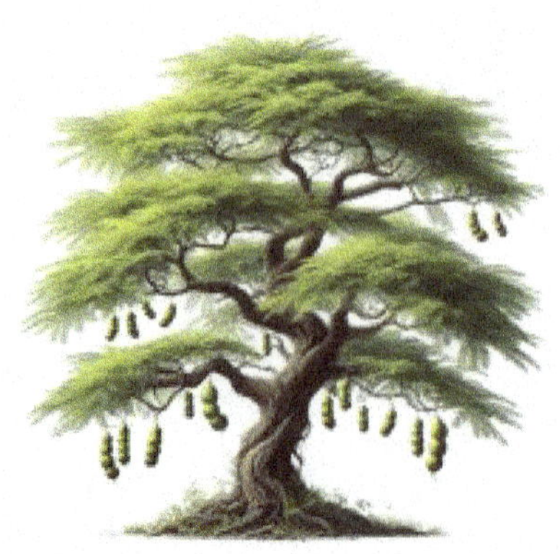

Tamarind Recipe:

Tamarind Roasted Vegetables

Ingredients:

3 sweet potatoes, peeled, cut into chunks

2 red bell peppers

2 yellow bell peppers

3 red onions, cut into wedges

1 large eggplant, cut into chunks

3 zucchinis, cut into thick chunks

4 tbsp sunflower oil

Tamarind paste:

1/2 cup (125ml) tamarind concentrate

1 lemongrass stem (white part only) finely chopped

3 garlic cloves, roughly chopped

2 tsp grated ginger

2 long red chiles, seeds removed, sliced

1 cup cilantro leaves

1/4 cup mint leaves, plus extra to garnish

2 tbsp honey

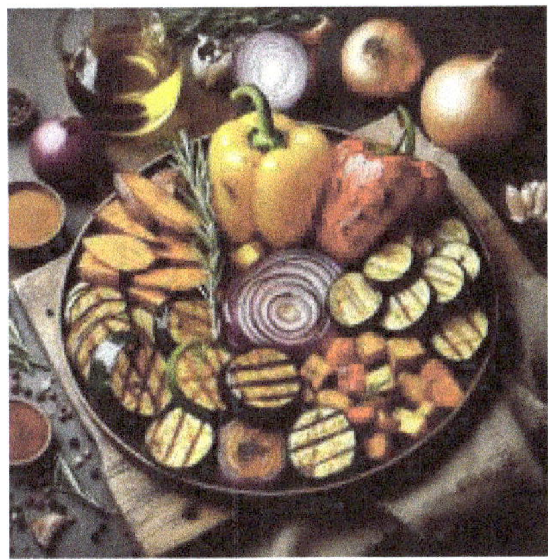

STEP 1

Preheat the oven to 190c/375f. For the tamarind paste, place all the ingredients in a food processor with 1/4 cup (60ml) boiling water. Blend to a thin paste, then set aside.

STEP 2

Toss the vegetables in the oil, spread over a large baking tray (you may need to use 2 trays depending on the size of your oven), then roast for 30 minutes. Remove from the oven and toss with the tamarind paste, then roast for a further 20-25 minutes until tender. Serve hot or at room temperature, garnished with the extra mint leaves.

Tamarind Nutritional Facts:

Tamarind Roasted Vegetables

Nutrition Facts

Servings: 2

Amount per serving

Calories 777

	% Daily Value*
Total Fat 29.9g	**38%**
Saturated Fat 3.1g	**15%**
Cholesterol 0mg	**0%**
Sodium 170mg	**7%**
Total Carbohydrate 125.3g	**46%**
Dietary Fiber 25g	**89%**
Total Sugars 64.1g	
Protein 14.3g	
Vitamin D 0mcg	0%
Calcium 224mg	17%
Iron 6mg	32%
Potassium 2774mg	59%

*The % Daily Value (DV) tells you how much a nutrient in a food serving contributes to a daily diet. 2,000 calorie a day is used for general nutrition advice.

Recipe analyzed

by **very**well

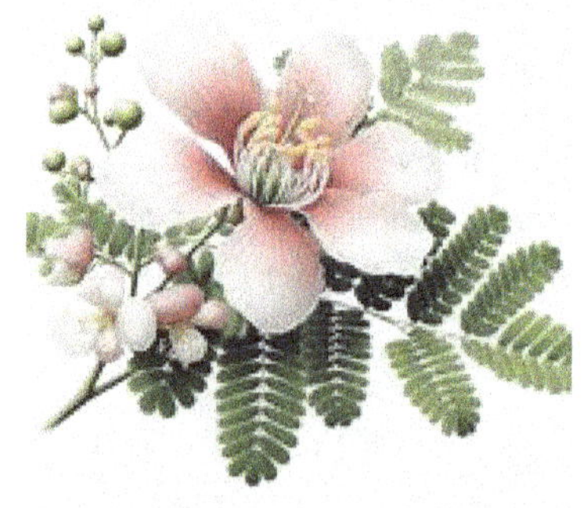

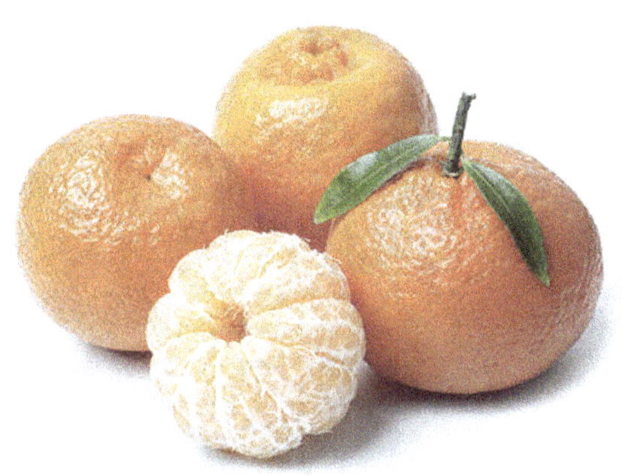

Tangerine: a type of citrus fruit that looks like small oranges with a tangy and sweet flavor.

They have a lot of fiber, vitamin C, and other nutrients that are good for your health.

You can eat tangerines fresh, squeeze them for juice, or use them as a garnish for salads.

The scientific name of tangerines is not clear. Some people consider them a separate species called Citrus tangerina, while others think they are a variety of mandarin orange (Citrus reticulata) or bitter orange (Citrus aurantium). The name was first used for fruit coming from Tangier, Morocco, described as a mandarin.

Tangerines are smaller and less round than oranges. The taste is considered less sour, as well as sweeter and stronger, than that of an orange. A ripe tangerine is firm to slightly soft, and pebble skinned with no deep grooves, as well as orange in color. The peel is thin, with a little bitter white mesocarp. Tangerines are mostly peeled and eaten by hand. The fresh fruit is also used in salads, desserts, and main dishes. The peel is used fresh, dried as a spice, or as a zest in baking and drinks.

Did you know that tangerines are also known for their health benefits? They are rich in vitamin C and antioxidants that help boost the immune system and protect against chronic diseases.

Tangerines are also an excellent source of thiamin, and folate. They contain naturally occurring sugars such as fructose, glucose, and sucrose. Tangerines also provide dietary fiber that is soluble, which helps slow digestion, stabilize blood glucose levels, and lower cholesterol.

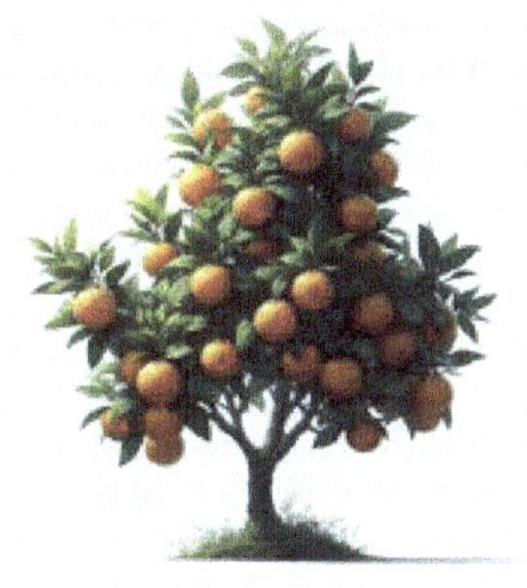

Tangerine Recipe:

Chile Tangerine Braised Lentils

Ingredients:

4 tbsp olive oil

1 carrot, finely chopped

1 onion, finely chopped

1 celery stick, finely chopped

2 red chiles, deseeded, finely chopped

2 garlic cloves, finely chopped

2 cups dried Puy lentils, rinsed

2 tbsp brown sugar

Juice of 6 tangerines, plus zest of 3

2 tbsp crème fraiche

1 bunch flat-leaf parsley, chopped

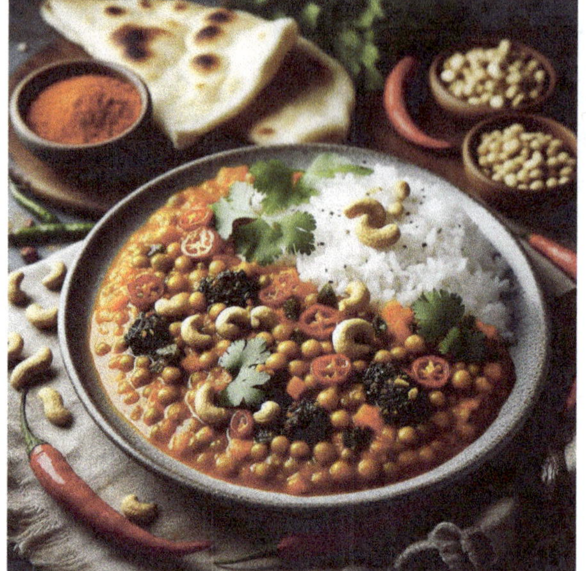

STEP 1

Heat the olive oil in a large saucepan. Add the carrot, onion, celery, chiles and garlic, and cook for 5-10 mins until the vegetables begin to soften. Add the rinsed lentils. Pour on two-thirds of the tangerine juice, then bring to the boil. Reduce the heat and simmer for 20-25 mins or until the lentils are tender and most of the liquid has been absorbed.

STEP 2

Remove from the heat and stir in the tangerine zest and remaining juice. Season with salt and pepper and allow to cool a little before stirring the crème fraiche and parsley. Serve warm or at room temperature.

Chile Tangerine Braised Lentils

Nutrition Facts

Servings: 6

Amount per serving

Calories	**522**

	% Daily Value*
Total Fat 23.6g	30%
Saturated Fat 1.5g	7%
Cholesterol 0mg	0%
Sodium 26mg	1%
Total Carbohydrate 53g	19%
Dietary Fiber 24.3g	87%
Total Sugars 6.7g	
Protein 21g	
Vitamin D 0mcg	0%
Calcium 72mg	6%
Iron 7mg	36%
Potassium 911mg	19%

*The % Daily Value (DV) tells you how much a nutrient in a food serving contributes to a daily diet. 2,000 calorie a day is used for general nutrition advice.

Recipe analyzed

verywell

by

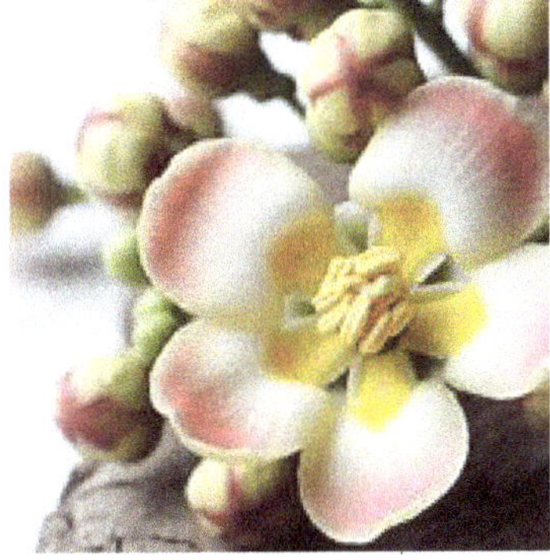

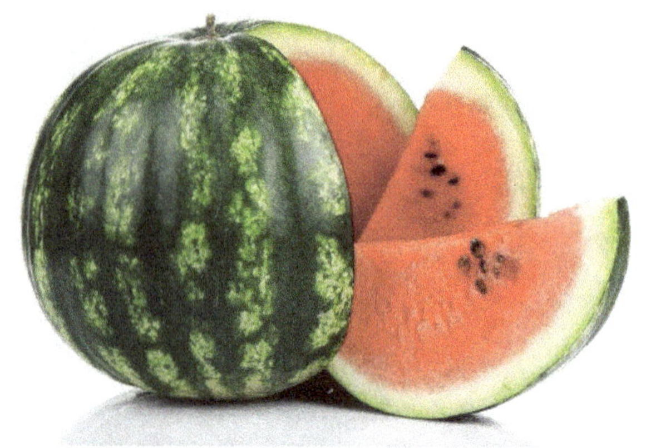

Watermelon: is a delicious and hydrating fruit that contains vitamins A and C, fiber, and water. These nutrients help support heart health, reduce muscle soreness, manage weight, aid digestion, and protect your skin. This fruit also has antioxidants such as lycopene and cucurbitacin E, which may have anticancer effects.

Watermelon can be enjoyed in many ways: fresh, in smoothies or juices, or as an ingredient for salads and other dishes. Watermelon is a low calorie and tasty summer treat that helps you stay hydrated while providing essential nutrients, including vitamins, minerals, and antioxidants.

Watermelons belong to the Cucurbitaceae family, along with cantaloupe, honeydew, and cucumber. There are five common varieties of watermelon: seeded, seedless, mini, yellow, and orange.

Here are some fun facts about watermelon:

Watermelons are made up of 92% water.

Watermelons are both a fruit and a vegetable.

You can eat the entire watermelon including the rind.

The world's heaviest watermelon weighed over 350 pounds.

Watermelons were used as canteens by early explorers in North America.

Watermelon Recipe:

Watermelon Smoothie

Ingredients:

½ cup watermelon, peeled and chopped

1 small banana, peeled and sliced

½ cup cold apple juice

 STEP 1 Blitz the watermelon in a blender with the banana and apple juice until smooth.

STEP 2 Pour the smoothie into a tall glass and serve immediately.

Enjoy this refreshing and healthy drink!

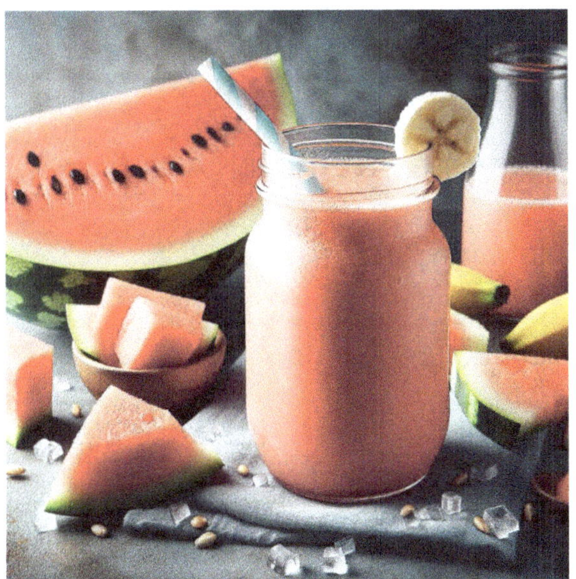

Watermelon Nutritional Facts:

Watermelon Smoothie

Nutrition Facts

Servings: 2

Amount per serving

Calories	**5717**
	% Daily Value*
Total Fat 15.3g	**20%**
Saturated Fat 5.1g	**26%**
Cholesterol 0mg	**0%**
Sodium 501mg	**22%**
Total Carbohydrate 1417.1g	**515%**
Dietary Fiber 26.6g	**95%**
Total Sugars 1210.7g	
Protein 11g	
Vitamin D 0mcg	0%
Calcium 1008mg	78%
Iron 9mg	52%
Potassium 12762mg	272%

*The % Daily Value (DV) tells you how much a nutrient in a food serving contributes to a daily diet. 2,000 calorie a day is used for general nutrition advice.

Recipe analyzed

by **very**well

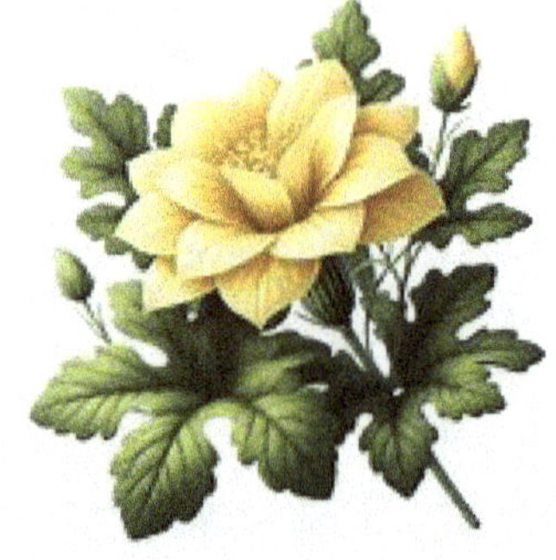